■ The 191 Best Practice-Building Strategies for Today's Physician

The Anthology of Tested and Proven Tactics From *The Practice Builder*, the Award-Winning Marketing Think Tank and Newsletter for Physicians

√ **W9-ARN-657**

■ The 191 Best Practice-Building Strategies for Today's Physician

The Anthology of Tested and Proven Tactics From *The Practice Builder,* the Award-Winning Marketing Think Tank and Newsletter for Physicians

■ Alan L. Bernstein, M.B.A.
With Donna Freiermuth

YEAR BOOK MEDICAL PUBLISHERS, INC.
CHICAGO • LONDON • BOCA RATON

1   2   3   4   5   6   7   8   9   0   E   R   92   91   90   89   88

Library of Congress Cataloging-in-Publication Data
Bernstein, Alan L.
    The 191 best practice-building strategies for today's physician.

    Includes bibliographies and index.
1. Medicine—Practice.   2. Medical care—Marketing.
I. Freiermuth, Donna P.   II. Practice builder.
III. Title.   IV. Title: One hundred ninety-one best
practice-building strategies for today's physician.
[DNLM: 1. Practice Management, Medical.   W 80 B531z]
R728.B443   1988   610'.68   87-23220
ISBN 0-8151-0720-X

Sponsoring Editor: Richard H. Lampert
Associate Managing Editor, Manuscript Services: Deborah Thorp
Copyeditor: Sally J. Jansen
Production Project Manager: Nancy Baker
Proofroom Supervisor: Shirley E. Taylor

*This is dedicated,
this is dedicated
to the one I love...
to the one I love.*

DIANA

■ PREFACE: WHAT'S REALLY INVOLVED IN BUILDING YOUR PRACTICE

☐ HOW TO USE THIS BOOK

Virtually every physician makes some effort to market and promote his or her practice. The promotion might be as understated as belonging to several local clubs and groups. But the fact remains that every doctor does some sort of marketing to promote his or her practice — regardless of whether it's labeled that or not.

The Practice Builder was created in response to today's increasingly competitive environment. It starts from the premise that astute professionals can no longer afford to ignore the growing competition they face. Instead, they need a source of ethical and effective strategies from which to choose. And by employing those strategies and tactics, they should not only survive but thrive.

Since its inception, *The Practice Builder* has become the most respected marketing think tank in the country. Strategies are explored, tested, and then fine-tuned only to be retested time and again. What is equally important, for every effective technique we discover we encounter at least ten times as many ineffectual strategies, even though they are often popular; examples abound in the marketplace.

This book is an anthology of those tested strategies and tactics for building a medical practice taken from issues of *The Practice Builder* newsletter.

As you read the articles in this and following chapters, keep a pencil in hand. Check the boxes beside articles with ideas you want to institute in your practice and make notes to yourself for later reference.

We hope that *The 191 Best Practice-Building Strategies for Today's Physician* is a source of fresh, profit-making ideas for you, so resist the temptation to read too quickly. Carefully consider the suggestions offered. If they don't seem appropriate to your situation at first glance, ask yourself what variations could make them suitable.

Dear *Practice Builder:*
I really feel like burying my head in the sand and wishing the competition just went away. But since they're here and I'm here and am going to compete, here's my concern: Can I really promote effectively *and* ethically at the same time?

A Concerned Practitioner

Dear Concerned:
Of course. Effectively means promising attractive results. And ethically means, in part, delivering what you promise. Together they mean repeat patients.
Gimmicks and half-truths may work once or twice, but people won't return. Patients have become too sophisticated. Today, you can't even fool some of the people some of the time.
Everyone should avoid deceptive practices. They almost always come back to haunt you through lawsuits or complaints to the Better Business Bureau or your medical association. They could even result in district attorney indictments.
Only ethical and effective promotion together can build a practice for the long run.

Sharing your concern,

Alan L. Bernstein
Publisher
The Practice Builder

■ MARKETING AIN'T ADVERTISING

When marketing is mentioned, most professionals think of advertising. An informal survey by G. Stanley Custer, M.D., past president of the American Group Practice Association, found this was the number 1 definition of marketing. Other common answers he uncovered: "Courteous, caring delivery of quality care;" and "courteous personnel and sufficient and clean washrooms."

Suffice it to say, marketing is a lot more. So Dr. Custer created an excellent working definition, one that integrates all the parts of the process:

- Marketing is proficient *research* into who and where the consumers in your service area are, and what their needs, wants, and preferences are.
- Developing quality service to meet those needs, wants, and preferences.
- Pricing them right.
- Making them convenient and accessible.
- Delivering them promptly at appropriate hours by courteous professionals and administrative personnel.
- Promoting those services by educating the public and providers and by creating awareness of those services by all means of communication in an ethical and professional manner.
- Finally, monitoring the results.

Notice that advertising doesn't come in until the mention of promoting and it would also include internal promotion, public relations, selling services directly to large organizations, and special events.

Look over the definition again carefully. Use it as a checklist for your own practice. If you find an element that you haven't integrated with your other marketing activities, rethink for a more complete plan—and for better profits.

☐ WHAT TO DO WHEN YOU DON'T LIKE MARKETING

At first, few professionals enjoy marketing themselves. Perhaps because the experience is new or, more likely, because we've been raised to think that self-promotion just isn't done. In either case, while your mind tells you that marketing is a key ingredient for success, your gut cries, "No!"

What to do? Unless you want to forget about marketing yourself and go to work for someone else, try this. Listen to your mind and ignore your gut. After your first winning effort, it'll take less intestinal fortitude the second time. And even less the next time.

You'll feel in control again.

☐ WORLD CLASS WINNERS

A study of Olympic athletes has a lesson for the professional: leading athletes aren't under great stress despite continued great challenges, because they feel in control of themselves. When loss comes, they're rarely devastated. Instead, they analyze their losses, looking for clues to improve future performance.

■ Ten Winning Ways to Explosive Growth

After all the excitement over the best-selling *In Search of Excellence*'s look at the traits of such well run behemoths as IBM and 3-M, Donald Clifford, Jr., of the management consulting firm of McKinsey and Co., took a close look at what the growth companies that are too small to make the *Fortune* 500 have in common.

These findings can be applied to an organization of any size—certainly to the medical professional practice—for explosive, targeted growth. Here are the winning ways that McKinsey and Company discovered:

Innovate as a way of life.—New services, new products, even new ways of doing business all combine to create an edge over the competition.

Compete on value, not price.—The winners deliver services that provide consistently superior value to all. Often these services cost more rather than less.

Develop a strong sense of mission.—The winners have an unusually clear sense of their distinctive role—where they'll compete and where they won't compete, the kinds of services they will and won't offer, the level of quality they expect to produce.

Attend to fundamentals.—Winners worry a lot about return on investment, strong financial disciplines, purchasing, measuring their performance, and hiring the best people.

Attack bureaucratization.—The winning companies consciously attack staff size.

Encourage experimentation.—Winners bend over backward not to punish failure, so that risk-takers have the freedom to make mistakes, learn from them, and generate new, more solid ideas.

Think like customers.—Winners have learned that the best way to make money for themselves is to fill their customers' needs beyond their expectations. They put themselves in their customers' shoes and also try to see through their customers' eyes. Their customers' concerns are truly their concerns.

Motivate with money.—Incentive pay tied to performance tends to be much higher in these winning companies than in ordinary organizations. A vested interest by employees proves itself again.

Set examples at the top.—The winning executives show extraordinary perseverance and are highly involved in the details of the organization. Their leaders are also people of vision. They want to build companies with values that transcend the mere creation of personal wealth. As one put it, "It's the inherent strength of my company and the way it's perceived by the community that is of greatest importance to me."

■ THE RIGHT AND WRONG WAY TO MAKE YOUR COLLEAGUES CRITICAL

Most professionals are concerned about what their colleagues think of them—and rightly so. So how do physicians maintain good colleague relationships while *effectively* building their practices? With great difficulty.

The trick is to make competitors feel threatened through excellent strategies, not angry at tactics that denigrate the image of the profession. Unfortunately, most promotions by doctors look like a year-end clearance at a discount furniture store. These retail-flavored, screaming promotions do nothing to enhance the credibility of medicine— especially since physicians and surgeons are under constant media fire.

When your promotion adds to the denigration, your colleagues will criticize you—with justification. But if you enhance the medical profession's image while reaping your own personal profits, no one can say "Peep." Only "I wish I'd done that."

■ CONTENTS

■ PART 1 Your Strategy: Strategic Thinking, Strategic Planning

■ CHAPTER 1
Where Do You Want To Be Tomorrow? How To Get There!

☐ YOUR MAP TO SUCCESS: THE ONE-PAGE MARKETING PLAN

Georgia physician K. M. wanted more patients beating a path to his door. So he'd been visiting the county library to study the ads in *Yellow Pages* directories from all over the country. He finally saw one that really appealed to him. He copied it and gave the half-page ad to his local directory publisher with instructions to reproduce it with his name at the bottom. Annual cost: $8,076.

The results? He made $5,120 in gross profit on $14,285 in income attributable to the *Yellow Pages* ad. After deducting the cost of the *Yellow Pages* ad, it left a loss of $2,956. The response had actually decreased over the previous year's smaller and less costly ad. K. M.'s mistake: Choosing an ad that was to his upwardly mobile liking, but not to the liking of his aging market's frugal needs. The ad simply looked too rich for their taste.

The Wrong Exit—That costly mistake is typical of practitioners first starting their marketing efforts. But the bigger mistake that underlies those errors is *a lack of planning*—not identifying the variables important to them and their practices and not realizing what must come first.

Trying to build your medical practice without a marketing plan makes as much sense as trying to find a distant city in an unfamiliar part of the country without figuring out the route to take. Without a map—the marketing plan—most practitioners get off the interstate before they reach the city. Many get off in the wrong state. Some even end up going around in circles. This lack of intelligent direction dooms most marketing efforts.

And the problem is only compounded when the practitioner asks directions from people who may not know enough to guide him— or worse—when he relies totally on someone with something to sell.

The Easy Way to the Right Exit—Your marketing plan saves you from getting lost or going around in circles by helping you to figure out the direction to go, the best route to take before you set out, *and which routes to avoid.*

While many advisers talk about the importance of a marketing plan, few professionals of any stripe have ever seen one. And fewer still know how to plot one.

To take the mystery out of marketing plans, *The Practice Builder* created the worksheet shown in Figure 1–1 and the following easy-to-follow guidelines for this most crucial of planning tools. To start, make several copies of both sides of the worksheet. Then as you read through the steps, jot down any ideas that come to you. Follow the step-by-step guidelines to get you thinking about how to produce your own one-page marketing plan that can chart your course for growth and to keep you on track. These steps are also discussed in great length in the remaining three chapters of this section.

1. *Define Your Objectives*: Define these for the short term—under 1 year. Then define them for the long term—more than 1 year. Express them in *a quantifiable and trackable way.* For example, 200 new patients within 6 months generating a total increase in revenues of $70,000; or increase recall percentage by ten points in next 6 months. If you don't quantify and track, you never know if you're succeeding or failing.

Caution! Practically all professionals automatically say "I'd like to double my practice." But it's not as simple as that. Step 7 will ask you how much you're willing to spend to achieve that goal. To play the game conservatively, figure that your budget must amount to 20% to 33% of your targeted increase in income to generate an equally conservative 333% to 500% return on investment.

And remember cash flow. Many strategies call for 50% to 75% of the marketing budget to be spent in the first 25% of the time. This usually means that first large chunk of cash needs to be in the bank at the start of the program, so it can't come out of expected cash flow.

2. *Identify Who Your Targets Are*: Define who you're trying to reach. Describe your target populations by their *chief* characteristics of age, sex, location, educational level, income, ethnicity/religion, blue collar vs. white collar, and life-style. Choose only those characteristics that

FIG 1–1.

Date _____

ONE-PAGE MARKETING PLAN WORKSHEET

1. **YOUR OBJECTIVE:**
   Short-term:
   Long-term:

2. **IDENTIFY YOUR TARGETS:**

   Age: Income:
   Sex: Education:
   Lifestyle: Location:
   White/Blue/"New" collar: Ethnicity/religion:
   Other:

3. **WHAT THOSE TARGETS WANT:**
   ___Experience ___Hours ___Location ___Price
   ___Other:

4. **WHO YOU ARE:**
   Location: Years of Experience:
   Credentials: Areas of Expertise:
   Strong Points: Weak Points:
   Honors/Awards: Practice Distinctions:
   Brief Description:

5. <u>MAIN COMPETITORS</u>:

    Name   Strengths   Weaknesses

   A.

   B.

   C.

   D.

6. <u>HOW TO COMPETE</u>:

   Primary Points:

   Secondary Points:

7. <u>DETERMINE YOUR BUDGET AND WHERE IT WILL COME FROM</u>:

8. <u>CHOOSE YOUR STRATEGY</u>:

   __Internal Promotion __*Yellow Pages* __Newspapers

   __Seminars __Public Relations __Others

   Specific Details:

9. <u>TIMING</u>:

   Important Considerations:

   Sequential Steps:

10. <u>EXECUTION</u>:

   Name   Responsibility   Date Due   Comments

   A.

   B.

   C.

   Where to start right now:

NOW BOIL DOWN BOTH SIDES OF WORKSHEET TO A ONE-PAGE
MARKETING PLAN. (Fig 1–2).

are important. Usually income, education, sex, age, and location are the most important factors. If you target business, describe it by industry, industry position, yearly sales, number of employees, and location.

Create a different one-page marketing plan for each target; for example, other practitioners from whom to generate referrals; senior citizens; blue-collar workers; 18- to 34-year-old females; and so on. Then order those groups by priority, targeting the easiest first.

3. *Define What the Targets Want:* What are the characteristics most important to the target group in selecting a physician in your field? Is it experience, hours, location, price?

4. *Define Who You Are:* What are your strengths? Weaknesses? What differentiates you in terms of your education, expertise, and years of experience? Credentials? What do you offer in terms of location, hours, pricing, equipment?

5. *Analyze Your Main Competitors:* Analyze just the ones you compete with in your normal trading area. But don't ignore the indirect competitors outside your profession to whom prospects could turn as a substitute, such as chiropractors, podiatrists, or psychologists. Chart each competitor's strengths and weaknesses.

6. *How to Compete*: How do you rate against those main competitors? Where can you best compete? List primary points. Then secondary points. Can you service your targets well or are you going too far outside of your area of expertise? Are you trying to draw from too far a distance? Or from a wealthier area from which you can't really attract? From across a mental market barrier that people won't usually cross—county lines, freeways, parkways or interstates, rivers, or large areas of open land?

Remember: Let's assume you have good, solid experience but one of your competitors has more. But if he or she doesn't promote experience and you do, you'll have that reputation for experience with the public. The same is true for any other advantage.

7. *Determine Your Budget*: How much are you willing to spend to accomplish the goal you spelled out in Step 1 above? How much can you afford now? Reconcile your budget with your goal.

8. *Choose Your Strategy*: Should it be internal promotion? *Yellow Pages*? Newspapers? Public relations? Seminars? Is the strategy you choose the most effective one? Weigh the pros and cons of different vehicles against each other.

9. *Choose Your Timing*: List events—both external to your practice and internal ones—that will affect your campaign over the time period specified in Step 1. Choose time of year, which months, what week to take action. Remember: If your practice has seasonal peaks, *promote heavily going into your busier periods*, not your practice lows. Your dol-

lars and efforts must work a lot harder in low periods when prospects aren't already looking for your services.

10. *Plan Your Execution:* Assign responsibilities. Set deadlines for all steps on a master time line.

Write the Marketing Plan Down—If you haven't done so yet, complete and polish your plan on a copy of the worksheet now. If your plan isn't in writing, it doesn't exist. By clarifying your thoughts on paper, you avoid your two greatest problems. First, being swayed by salespeople into buying inappropriate or useless promotion. And, second, failing to consider all the important variables that will in turn produce less than optimal results or often no results at all.

Now boil your ideas down to fit the one page plan in Figure 1–2. You'll find that under each of the ten headings, there are only two or three important ideas. Unless you limit your plan to one page, too many extraneous variables will dilute your concentration. So focus only on the important ones. The marketing plans that follow are examples of ones that different physicians would create for themselves.

Now you're ready to boost your practice and increase your earnings with confidence. It's this planning that invariably separates the super successes who reach their goals from the horror stories who were sidetracked and never got near their destination.

If you fail to plan, then plan to fail.

☐ SAMPLE MARKETING PLAN: REACTIVATING A PSYCHIATRIST'S PATIENTS

1. Objective: Add 10 billable hours per week.
2. Target: Inactive patient base.
3. What targets want: To feel happy, content, fulfilled; to solve problems.
4. Who you are: A 42-year-old psychiatrist, 12 years in practice in Atlanta, emphasizing clinical practice; practice is at 70% capacity. Have about a thousand inactive files.
5. Main competitors: None for this target market.
6. How to compete: Remind former patients that if they're feeling unhappy or troubled now, they need not. Since they've learned some of the basics on how to turn their lives around, perhaps all they need is some short-term assistance to get them back on track. If they can't do it themselves, suggest that they contact my office. Tell them the time frame is usually short for patients who have been in therapy before.
7. Budget: $500.

FIG 1–2.

Date_____

ONE-PAGE MARKETING PLAN

1. YOUR OBJECTIVE:
   Short-term:
   Long-term:

2. IDENTIFY YOUR TARGETS:

3. WHAT THOSE TARGETS WANT:

4. WHO YOU ARE:

5. MAIN COMPETITORS:
     Name   Strengths   Weaknesses

     A.
     B.
     C.
     D.

6. HOW TO COMPETE:

7. DETERMINE YOUR BUDGET AND WHERE IT WILL COME FROM:
8. CHOOSE YOUR STRATEGY:

9. TIMING:

10. EXECUTION:

8. Strategy: Write a two-page letter on office stationery to inactive patients. Start with a case history to illustrate the point. Then explain why they should return if they're having problems. Avoid sounding self-serving. Write a second letter with a different illustration, same point. Mail second package 90 days later.

9. Timing: Write letters by October 20. Print bids by November 2. Hire mailing house to stuff and bulk mail using postage meter by November 7. Have printing completed by November 10. Mail first package on November 20. Mail second package on April 10.

10. Execution: I write letters; secretary to type and get print bids and select mailing house. I supervise printing and mailing as well.

☐ SAMPLE MARKETING PLAN: CHANGING LOCATION

1. Objective: Increase new patients by 50% within 12 months.

2. Target: 25 to 50 years old, 65% blue collar, 60% female, within a 4-mile radius.

3. What target wants: Quality care.

4. Who you are: General practitioner, 2 years in practice, located in professional building with very little foot traffic.

5. Main competitors: Eight general and family physicians.

6. How to compete: Give office much greater exposure and greater convenience.

7. Budget: $22,000.

8. Strategy: Change location to new shopping center under construction. Locate between incoming supermarket with its high-volume foot traffic (65% female) and sports and fitness center with its 1,000 members. Promote to sports center members with seminars at the club and articles in their newsletter. Promote to all traffic in the shopping center with outdoor office signs—on the front, side, and back of mall. Use the signs to position office as convenient for checkups, inoculations, standard tests, family care.

9. Timing: Move in 4 months. Start sign design in 1 month. Approach sports and fitness center in 1 month to explore seminars and articles.

10. Execution: I choose sign design within 30 days; I deal directly with sports and fitness center, landlord, and contractor. The office manager coordinates the move. (With scarce resources, *only* spend on immediate income producers, like signs and sports center promotion.) Finish final inside amenities with future income.

☐ SAMPLE MARKETING PLAN: PROMOTING WITHIN A PPO OR IPA

1. Objective: Increase professional referrals, especially from fellow PPO and IPA panel docs.

2. Target: Nonreferring primary care physicians from PPOs and IPAs, as well as other GPs, FPs, OB/GYNs and pediatricians in the area.

3. What target wants: To refer to an expert whose care will reflect back favorably on them.

4. Who you are: 44-year-old ear, nose and throat specialist, 5 years in suburban Louisiana, relocated from successful practice in Massachusetts. Conservative in promotion.

5. Main competitors: Six other ENTs in immediate area.

6. How to compete: Differentiate myself by informing prospective referrers of my expertise so they'll view me as the authority.

7. Budget: $3,500 over 12 months.

8. Strategy: Write and mail quarterly newsletter on breakthroughs and important information for primary care physicians to know about ENT. Use high-line image. Write short articles using many examples of cases I've cured. From these, make the general point of each article. Mention membership in PPOs and IPAs. Mention any talks, articles, or interviews I'm doing.

Format: 11x17-in. glossy paper folded to $8^{1}/_{2}$x11-in.; two colors; mailed flat in 9x12-in. envelope. For extra response, follow up with phone call after each issue to ask for their questions, comments, and a lunch meeting.

9. Timing: Hire graphic artist to design newsletter by April 1. Write first issue by same date. Have issue laid out for printer by April 15. Compile and computerize mailing list by April 15. Mail first issue on May 1. I start follow-up calls by May 7.

10. Execution: I write and edit each issue; I hire a graphic artist to design it and lay out each issue. I have Jane type issues. I compile mailing list; Jane enters it on the computer and oversees mailing. I make follow-up calls.

☐ SAMPLE MARKETING PLAN: PUBLIC SEMINARS

1. Objective: 40 radial keratotomy (RK) surgeries per month at $3,000 per case for the next 12 months. Total RK income: $1,440,000.

2. Target: 25- to 45-year-olds; 65% are female and in middle to upper income bracket, insured by specific companies who cover RK.

3. What target wants: To be unencumbered by glasses or contacts; to see well; to look attractive.

4. Who you are: Board-certified ophthalmologist, 6 years in practice, centrally located.

5. Main competitors: Three other ophthalmologists doing RK. But the real competition is continued use of glasses or contacts.

6. How to compete: Educate targets about benefits, efficiency, and safety of RK.

7. Budget: $200,000.

8. Strategy: Conduct public seminars in top-line hotels to explain RK. Use slides that emphasize benefits and results. Use patient testimonials (check state regulations). Promote seminars heavily in newspaper and by direct mail to upper-middle income areas. Emphasize to members of the audience that if they're insured by certain companies, all or part of the cost is covered. Financing is also available. Have all ads, mail packages, and seminar materials professionally prepared.

9. Timing: Hire ad agency within 2 weeks to prepare materials. Set newspaper ads and direct mail to break in 8 weeks for first seminar scheduled in 10 weeks. Schedule two seminars per month.

10. Execution: Ad agency is responsible for promotion. I supervise it. The office manager is responsible for seminar logistics. I give the seminars. Agency prepares seminar materials.

☐ SAMPLE MARKETING PLAN: HEALTH FAIR

1. Objective: Talk to 200 people in 2 days at a local health fair, and attract five new cosmetic surgery patients. Increase awareness of practice to increase *Yellow Pages* response and word-of-mouth referrals.

2. Target: Community residents; primary markets—females, 25 to 55 years old and at least middle income. Secondary market—males, executives, aged 40 years or older.

3. What target wants: Beauty, recognition.

4. Who you are: Cosmetic surgeon, board-certified, 11 years experience.

5. Main competitors: Seven non–board-certified cosmetic surgeons, none of whom will be at the health fair.

6. How to compete: Position yourself as *the* specialist in the community. Create exciting booth.

7. Budget: $600.

8. Strategy: Make booth highly visible and information intensive. Use large photos to catch the eye and show the beauty achieved by RK. Also use big headlines about beauty and offer information and

☐ Top Consultant Reveals Way to Achieve 25% Growth

When it comes to quantifying your goal as described in Step 1 of the marketing plan, Ira Maser,[1] well-known management consultant and president of MGMT International, says star performers work with a dollar goal. From it, Maser explains, they're able to figure how many patients they must see each day or week and how much the average prospect must spend. From there, they devise the overall strategies and specific tactics to get to those numbers.

Star performers break their case and production goals down to a daily or weekly basis. Then they write them down. And they *carry* these figures with them while working.

"With an objective measure of your daily and weekly performance with you, you know exactly where you stand," Maser said. "And in every case I've seen, the professional works more efficiently, much smarter, and makes more money."

---

free consultation right then and there. To increase responses, assistants will *ask* passersby if they would like information. I will examine, consult, and make recommendations; the assistant offers to schedule an in-office appointment for the next week and gives office literature and appointment card; the front desk will reconfirm appointments by phone. Assistants take every person's name and address for office mailing list.

9. Timing: Order additional literature 6 weeks ahead of time. Hire a graphic artist 8 weeks ahead of time to design show-stopping booth graphics with an ultraprofessional look and image.

10. Execution: I'll choose the graphic designer to design the booth. In my office Donna coordinates setup, personnel, scheduling, and other booth details. I conduct a run-through 2 days before the fair.

☐ WHAT MARKETING NUMBERS YOU SHOULD KNOW

Motivational speakers are fond of stories like the one about the physician whose friends would ask him, "Are you rich yet?" In the beginning of his practice, he'd answer, "No, not yet." As the years went on, when they'd ask again, and he would still answer, "No, not yet." Even after he'd earned the first million. And the second.

Throughout his life, he never did feel rich. Unfortunately, he died at 51 years of age. Certainly it didn't have to be this way, because all he had to do was to define what "rich" is. Most of us would probably agree that having a half a million dollars in investments is comfortable; having a million is rich; having 2 million is ultrarich. Had he done this, he might have been able to enjoy it.

Is Your Marketing "Rich?"—In marketing, we need to use numbers in the same way. If we don't know the numbers that measure performance, we don't know what's working, if anything. We don't know which effort is losing so we can change or drop it. And if we don't set goals and define expectations, we don't know if the promotion is rich or poor.

Here are the common marketing numbers to be concerned about. Not knowing them makes you anxious. Knowing them gives you control.

1. *Average Case Size*: This is the average gross number of dollars generated by the average new patient during the first 12 months he or she is with you. It doesn't include income from referrals or second year visits but does reflect repeat visits during the first year. It's a good yardstick for income to be expected from a new patient within a reasonable period of time.

But more than that, it tells you how much you can spend to generate a new patient. If new patients bring in an average of $1,000 per year, you can spend $50, $200, $400, even $500 to get one good qualified case. If case size runs $400, you'll lower your expenditure parameters. This figure also lets you tell your accountants they're wrong when they recite the usual rule of thumb that you should limit your promotional expenditure to $25 per new patient. It's usually not enough and has no relationship to the income to be generated. Determine your average case size by pulling every tenth chart from last year's new patients, add up the gross income, and divide by the number of cases.

2. *Old Dollars vs. New Dollars:* Of last year's gross dollars, how many came from existing patients and how many from new ones? How does this compare to the year before? By knowing this, you'll know whether to pay more attention to reaching out to the community for new patients or developing better internal marketing to improve retention. For each practice, there's an optimal balance. Find yours by pulling a random sample of charts and adding up the new and old dollars.

3. *Responses by Promotion:* Source code each promotion. Use a fictitious phone extension or a fictitious receptionist's name ("Ask for Elizabeth") to key where and when the promotion appeared. Keep a tally sheet next to the phone. When the appointment is made, also put the key next to the name in the appointment book and in the chart. Total the new patients generated by the different promotions.

4. *Return on Investment:* The number of respondents is insufficient information by itself. But it's needed to get the *only* statistic that's really meaningful—return on investment, which is how many dollars came in from a source divided by the cost of that promotion. Was it 300%? Or 500% Or 5%? Less than 100% means you lost money.

If you don't calculate the return on investment and just rely on the number of respondents to a promotion, you could have 50 respondents, yet each one only spent an average of $60 when the promotion cost $3,560. That amounts to a loss of $560. Or you might dismiss a promotion that only resulted in five responses unless you tally the revenue. The five cases could have totaled $13,700 in revenue at a cost of only $2,200. That's a return on investment of 622%.

5. *Recall Percentage:* And how successful are your recalls? Without knowing what percent responds to your efforts, you don't know how much you need to constantly turn to external marketing to replace the patients who don't return to you over time, or whether you need to work on your recall system more. Unless you take the time and effort to calculate these various marketing numbers, you don't know whether you're very rich—or headed for the poorhouse.

REFERENCE

1. Interview with Ira Maser. MGMT International (10880 Wilshire Boulevard, Suite 1007, Los Angeles, CA 90024).

■ CHAPTER 2
Who's Most Likely To Need You: Marketing With A Precision Rifle, Not A Shotgun

☐ HOW TO SEGMENT YOUR MARKET

Most professionals intuitively understand that the market for their services doesn't include everyone. Selective marketing, rather than a shotgun approach, means a better return on your investment. But how can you define your market so you can deal with it efficiently?

Defining The Market—Psychiatrist S.A. has the answer. She defines her primary market as middle- to upper-income males and females who are 25 to 45 years old, living in a wealthy Southern California coastal community, and under great work-related stress. And they're ready to be helped. Hence, her local *Yellow Pages* directory carries her ad, augmented by elegant graphics, that reads: "Professionals only. Exclusively for men and women in high-stress positions within the executive, management, and professional community. Depression. Marital or family problems. Sexual dysfunction. Sleep disturbance. Complete confidentiality."
Since people earning a high income define themselves as "professional," the ad nicely qualifies prospects by their ability to pay.

Market Categories—Philip Kotler, the Harold T. Martin Professor of Marketing at Northwestern University, Chicago, explains the process. In his book *Marketing for Nonprofit Organizations*,[1] Kotler lists the ways to describe prevalent markets today. The markets are broken down under the major geographic, demographic, or psychographic/motivational categories.

1. Describe your market geographically: Generally, the geographic category means you target your market as the target population within an "X"-mile radius of your office. But in defining that radius, several factors should be taken into account:

- Population density—urban/suburban/rural. The lower the density, the greater the radius and therefore the greater the area you should encompass.
- Physical barriers such as mountains and lakes, affect the area from which you can attract business.
- Mental barriers that also affect a prospect's buying behavior include county lines, major roads, stretches of open or undeveloped land, or poorer neighborhoods. Prospects are unlikely to cross these mental barriers so your radius should reflect these barriers (see sidebar).

2. Describe your market demographically:

- By age: Under 6 years old; 6 to 11; 12 to 17; 18 to 34; 35 to 49; 50 to 64; over 64.
- By sex.
- By family size: one- or two-person families; those with three or four members; over five members.
- By family life cycle: young, single; young married or cohabiting, no children; young married, youngest child under 6 years old; young married, youngest child 6 years old or older; older married with no children under 18 years old; older single.
- By income: under $9,999; $10,000 to $19,999; $20,000 to $29,999; $30,000 to $49,000; $50,000 + .
- By occupation: professionals and technicians; managers, officials, and proprietors; clerical workers and salespersons; craftspeople, foremen, and operators; farmers; retired persons; students; housewives; unemployed persons.
- By education: grade school or less; some high school; high school graduates; some college; college graduates.
- By religion: Catholic; Protestant; Jewish; other.
- By race: white; black; Asian; other.
- By ethnicity/nationality: Mexican-American; Latin American; Italian-American; Irish-American; German-American; Japanese-American; Middle Eastern immigrants; Eastern European immigrants; and so on.
- By social class: lower-lower; upper-lower; lower-middle; middle-middle; upper-middle; and so on.
- Targeting business: number of employees; annual sales; industry; industry ranking; sole owner/partnership/corporation; local/regional/national/international.

☐ Mental Barriers?

A good example of mental barriers comes from the experience of podiatrist T.W. He bought a practice that had been barely making it. He hoped to double that practice within 18 months through a big promotional plan. The plan: to promote in a retirement community about 6 miles away. With over 1,000 residents and only one competing podiatrist near them, he felt that with a promotional blitz, he could corral most of the injured feet into his office.

He began by writing a column for the community newspaper. Then he gave four talks in the community in 2-months' time. A direct mail piece followed that made no offer but created strong name recognition—a solid program.

Results: dismal. A few hearty souls hobbled out to his office, but most went to the competing podiatrist near their community who also promoted his practice heavily.

Unseen Boundaries.—The problem was market barriers. Most people won't cross certain boundaries to do their shopping, whether it's for clothing or health services. Some of these boundaries are physical barriers that define natural markets such as rivers, hills or mountains, lakes, and so on. But most barriers are mental.

Distance is the foremost barrier. In urban markets, about 90% of one's patients come from within a mile and a half of the practice. In suburban markets, it's 3 to 4 miles. There are a great many exceptions to the rule, but T.W.'s practice wasn't one of them. In his suburban market only the dedicated made the effort.

Remember: Where seniors, children, animals, or repeat visits are concerned, trading areas tend to be smaller.

Socioeconomic Barriers.—Also potent as a barrier are socioeconomic boundaries. Oftentimes, physicians in middle-income areas would like to attract a pocket of the wealthy only a mile or two away. Save your time and money. By and large, people in a higher income area won't buy in a lower income one.

Other mental barriers.—Large expanses of open land make people think the world stops there. County lines do also, even if the prospect is little further than across the street. Parkways, freeways, and turnpikes sometimes have the same effect.

Can you overcome these market barriers? Yes, but usually the price is too high for a minimal return. T.W. overcame his market barrier by opening a satellite office in the main medical complex that served the retirement village. Due to his earlier and continuing promotion, it was an immediate success. "I suspected that it might be a little hard to attract the prospects I wanted, but the resistance was unbelievable. It was an expensive lesson."

3. Describe your market psychographically/motivationally:
- By life-style: swinger; status seeker; plain Joe; family oriented; and so forth.
- By personality: compulsive; gregarious; conservative; ambitious; and so on.
- By benefits sought: economy; convenience; quality; dependability; prestige; reduction of fear; and so on.
- By user status: nonuser of a service or product; potential user; first-time user; regular user; ex-user.
- By usage rate: light user; medium user; heavy user. (Brewers know that 80% of beer is drunk by 20% of beer drinkers. They market accordingly.)
- By loyalty status: none; medium; strong; absolute.
- By readiness stage: unaware; vaguely aware; informed; interested; intending to buy.

Pinpoint Variables—According to Dr. Kotler, you should identify the most important variables in describing your segments of the market. Not all apply. Work with the major ones. For instance, an orthopedic surgeon could pinpoint middle- and upper middle-class school-aged children who participate in sports and gymnastics living within a 10-mile radius.

Such segmenting helps you choose the most appropriate media, write the promotional copy, design new services, adjust pricing, determine payment methods, and even select your office staff.

Defining your markets allows you to put yourself in your prospective patients' shoes and identify with their needs. And that is the essence of marketing.

☐ WHEN THE MARKET TALKS, ARE YOU LISTENING?

As we've seen, closely defining your market lets you put yourself in your patients' shoes. But understanding their needs also means actively listening to their concerns and preferences. It applies to individual practitioners as well as an entire specialty. A good example of the need to truly listen to your patients was the experience of obstetricians and hospitals in the 1970s.

In the face of a growing preference for less drugged childbirths on the part of young expectant parents, many obstetricians and hospitals continued to prefer to do business as they had always done it—traditional childbirths in the cold environment of the delivery room. Those physicians and the hospitals who refused to recognize that maternity patients had a legitimate say in whether drugs should be administered in a normal delivery and what the setting should be found their case load dwindling. Instead, expectant mothers sought out obstetricians and hospitals who recognized those concerns and addressed them without compromising the quality of care they offered.

Perspective Problems—The obstetricians who saw their patient base shrink ran into trouble from where they were starting out. They tried to get prospects to do what they wanted rather than what the patient wanted. They failed to listen to their prospects and, instead, were only concerned with telling them what they thought the expectant mother needed. While their concern for safe deliveries certainly played a part, some of the resistance was a preference for the familiar or for the status quo, an aversion to listening to what the patient wants.

Any market behaves like huge waves moving toward the shore. A practitioner is powerless to channel them in another direction. But to harness the power, you can flow in the same direction while still practicing good medicine, drawing patients to you as you go, and enjoying the process.

☐ IDENTIFYING WITH YOUR MARKET: HOW TO AND HOW NOT TO

One caution should be made about identifying with your patients. Professionals who call *The Practice Builder* advisory hotline occasionally object to a recommended strategy. Typically they'll say, "Knowing what I know, if I were choosing a professional, I wouldn't be influenced by that strategy." The pitfall is that practitioners aren't representative of the patients who use their services. They're *too sophisticated* a consumer, with concerns that aren't shared by the typical prospective patient.

Rather than view your services by taking into account the wealth of knowledge you have about your field, place yourself in the mindset of your typical patient. Rarely are they overly sophisticated about your services, and many times they're first-time buyers. Write down their concerns, and create your strategies directly from there.

☐ THE STRATEGY CORNER: BREADTH, DEPTH, OR MARKET SHARE

Any tack you use to expand a practice boils down to one of three basic growth strategies. It amounts to expansion by breadth, depth, or market share. After exploring each of those expansion strategies and analyzing its advantages and pitfalls, we'll dissect some of the proven ways to put each into practice.

■ Expanding Your Market's Breadth

Reaching Out—In essence, expanding the breadth of the market means bringing in new patients who have never before bought *your professional or specialty's* services. For the cosmetic surgeon, it's men. For the allergist, it's those who might not suspect they have an allergy.

Sound difficult? It is. In fact, of the three basic strategies, expanding the breadth of a market is the hardest. Why? Because consumers are most resistant to a service or product they've never used before.

Over and Over—The way to overcome that resistance? Tell them why they need your service. But more importantly, tell them over and over again. Repetition is the key. Few people respond the first time they're told of a new service or product. But the more they hear of or see it, the more familiar and comfortable they feel—and the more likely they are to seek the service. That's why the more promotion you do, the more effective it becomes.

The problem is that repeating the message necessary to bring someone new into the marketplace is expensive. So this type of strategy is best done on a cooperative basis.

National and state associations or large private groups can pool resources to get the job done—assuming, of course, they want to, and you can get enough participants to agree on need, strategy, tactics, budget, timing, and other factors. Judging from the meager, ineffective attempts made, professional associations find this hard to accomplish.

New Approach—In reality, it takes a different organization to tackle this strategy, one created specifically for this purpose. It's a promotional co-op that brings together practitioners into a group to promote the benefits of their specialty's services to nonusers.

Begin by selecting practitioners who don't compete by virtue of their location. Pool your resources to advertise in mass media or to sell your services as a unit to corporations, unions, PPOs, IPAs, or insurance companies. Either way, make sure you direct the business generated to participating professionals, perhaps by a central referral phone number.

Since repetition takes time, all participants must commit to supporting the group for a definite and sufficiently long term. Use a tightly written *contract* and a *promissory note* to assure that everyone acts in concert and remains committed.

Use an Expert—Since it's absolutely impossible to create good promotion by committee, hire an expert to produce the promotional materials. Use as small a committee as possible—preferably three or fewer—to approve materials and give guidance, not to write the copy or to create.

It's possible, however, to attract new buyers into a market all by yourself—but only under certain circumstances. To make up for the restricted resources and repetition, you must have a new procedure or product that only you offer—perhaps a unique procedure.

Another way is to promote a new development in your field that many practitioners offer, but one that isn't well known to the public. Simply be the only professional in your area publicizing that new capability. That implies that prospects should come only to you. A good example of this in ophthalmology is radial keratotomy (RK). Many ophthalmologists now have the capability, but few make the development known to nonusers or to those who have no knowledge about RK.

In any event, this strategy is tough at best and requires big dollars, an extremely unique proposition, or a quick promotional campaign to capitalize on an industry breakthrough. But if you win, you win big.

■ Expanding Your Market's Depth

Unlike breadth expansion, expanding depth is much easier, less costly, and has little risk. In this market strategy, you focus on filling more of your existing patients' needs. It's much easier to have a current patient buy services rather than trying to convince someone with whom you have no established relationship to buy your services.

But be careful. This is not a prescription to overprescribe. That would not only be unethical but would also destroy patient confidence, greatly damaging your practice in the long run.

More Complete Care—Expanding your market's depth is the thorough identification of all of your patients' needs through skillful investigation along with the development of additional capabilities to provide more complete care.

There are two ways to discover new needs: (1) Take the time to engage your most promising patients in a detailed discussion, asking probing questions to uncover needs they're not aware of. The time required to probe deeply is the drawback, but it's extremely productive with high-potential prospects. (2) Help educate your patients to identify their own needs. Feed them information. Use brochures in your waiting room. Send out quarterly newsletters or other periodic mailings. Or use a "1-minute message" as described in Chapter 6. Results: Immediate sales of that service will increase. Referrals for that service will also increase. And because of the residual effects, you'll receive requests for that service up to a year later.

New Services—There are also two ways to expand your offerings of new services: (1) Add services in demand. For generalists this could mean undertaking more specialty work rather than referring those cases out. And for specialists, it could mean adding new state-of-the-art procedures to keep well ahead of the inevitable encroachment by generalists. (2) Inform your present patients and the public of those new offerings—tastefully, convincingly, and repeatedly. How?

Here, again, use the 1-minute message to spread the word. Follow up with a postcard mailing to patients announcing the new services. Postcards carry a sense of urgency, especially when you begin your copy with "Instead of waiting for our normal mailing, I felt you needed to know about our new _____ right away."

If you have a practice newsletter, make the new services the subject of your lead article, or write two or three articles about different aspects of the services. In fact, dedicate the entire issue to announcing the services. There's no room for modesty—just effectiveness.

Better yet, since people always read personalized, first-class mail, tell them your news in a package they're sure to notice.

Inactive Files—Also use your new services to recall patients you know would personally profit. Write a special letter, or have your front desk call to explain the benefits personally.

Remember:

1. Face-to-face is the most powerful form of communication, followed in order by telephone, first-class mail and news stories, then third-class bulk mail, including newsletters. Use the most powerful form you can afford.

2. People can't take advantage of your new abilities if they don't know about them.

3. People are reluctant to buy until they feel comfortable with the concept—which means telling them repeatedly.

Expanding the depth of your market is much easier and less costly than expanding the breadth of your market and has little risk. Depth expansion helps your bottom line, but it doesn't necessarily expand your new patient count. For that, look to your market share.

■ Expanding Your Market Share

In market-share expansion, you grow by attracting dissatisified patients of competing practitioners or other professionals' satisfied patients to whom you offer more attractive benefits: You're faster, better, less expensive, or whatever. This strategy is the true essence of competition.

Tactics—Differentiate yourself from seeming look-alikes. Often practitioners believe their practice may not be any different from many others. Just as no two people are completely alike, no two practices are either. The trick is to identify those differences. And to make them meaningful to prospective patients.

The Crucial Step—Communicate your differences. Patients of competing practices won't switch without convincing and repetitive messages.

☐ OFFERING WHAT PEOPLE REALLY WANT

According to the *Missouri Motivational Study,* professionals are wrong four out of five times about what their patients and clients really want. The study showed that people value the effort expended six times more than the results. That concern ranked second and competence third was also interesting. So be energetic. And show it.

Your 9-to-5 office hours are seldom really convenient except to patients who don't have jobs to go to. What we often forget is that working has become the norm for the vast majority of both men and women. Research has now established that there's no adult at home during the workday in seven out of ten American homes. For that reason, rethink the hours you offer your services.

Test one night a week and/or every other Saturday morning. If the time gets booked, expand it slowly. Add associates cautiously for expanded business.

If the test time gets booked but it's merely a redistribution of existing business, not an increase, consider expanding the evening/weekend hours and reducing weekdays. Reason: Convenience keeps your patients in the long run.

☐ MARKETING TO THE NEW-COLLAR CLASS

We've all heard of white collar and blue collar—even those so poor that they've been labeled the "no collars." But those broad brush

How to Know Where to Spend Your Promotional Budget

In taking all these factors into account when defining your geographic market, one final caution is not to overlook an area from which you can draw.

There are a variety of reasons why people in certain communities come to you but residents of other areas don't. A zip code analysis allows you to identify all the neighborhoods from which you are currently attracting patients. It will also allow you to spot the areas that you haven't been able to penetrate for whatever reason.

The Analysis—On a zip code map of your region, place a different color pin for each of your patients. For example, use blue pins for active patients, white ones for those seen in the last 2 years, and red for those not seen in more than 2 years. Then analyze your distribution and your growth.

This will allow you to better target your promotional budget and activities. Focus your direct mail campaign on specific zip codes to double up your returns. Cultivate organizations in areas where you're already popular with speaking engagements. And check whether your advertising media reach into those communities you really want to target.

Results: A.F., a suburban Chicago physician, literally had five different local *Yellow Pages* directories in which he could place his display ad. With a limited budget, he knew he should choose only two of them. His zip code analysis clearly ranked the five areas for him. Picking the two that were most cost-effective then became simple. "In fact, my analysis showed that the third-ranking area was almost as profitable as my second. So I decided to increase my budget and include my ad in that area's directory. If I hadn't analyzed my data, I would certainly have picked at least one wrong area."

---

strokes are too wide to describe a distinctively different group of people with their own buying behavior.

The new-collar class consists of those individuals who are *highly educated* with anywhere from 2 to 6 years of post-high school training. They include teachers, nurses, administrative assistants, pharmacists, low-level management, and the like. But they *don't* have a lot of money. Income levels may range from $20,000 to $40,000. Add family responsibilities, and it's tight.

So the trademark of this large class of prospects is their well–thought-out buying decisions that emphasize value. This is different from the designer-label focus of yuppies and different from the ultraquality, price-is-no-object concerns of the professional class. It also differs from the lowest income groups' emotionally responsive buying of minimal quality goods and services as well as the less-educated buying decisions of the blue-collar trade, although this last group is also value conscious. No, this is a different group, and its wears a different collar—a "new collar."

How to Market to the New Collar—Since enduring quality and good pricing are paramount to this group, that is what the promotional message must contain—quality and affordability. That means lots of credentials, claims of experience, expertise, specialization, high technology, and a high level of caring—but at an attractive price.

Because of the emphasis on value and price, the new-collar market responds well to loss-leader advertising whereby a low price is offered for a service to attract new prospects who then buy other services at your regular fees. When a GP charges $25 for checkups, the patients that come in with big cases are either new collar or blue collar. The "no collars" make up the remainder and must be sifted through to get to the highly desirable patients. (For profit maximization in loss-leader advertising, keep fees high on all non–price-sensitive services.)

New-collar promotion must make the claim of affordability. But to do this, price *need not* be mentioned. Certainly, price promotion enhances and proves the claim. Therefore it generates more response. However, the claim of affordability alone, with the embellishment of how you believe high-quality services should be within the reach of all discerning people, often suffices.

Remember: This highly intelligent, price-conscious group is large—much larger than the yuppies and upper-middle class that most physicians seek. So gear your message appropriately if your target is wearing a new collar.

REFERENCE

1. Kotler P: *Marketing for Non-Profit Organizations*, Englewood Cliffs, NJ, Prentice-Hall Inc, 1982, p 105.

■ CHAPTER 3
Defining You Vs. Them: Who's A Colleague;
Who's A Competitor

☐ **LEADING EXPERT EXPLAINS FORMULA FOR PRACTICE SUCCESS: AN INTERVIEW WITH D. L. SOLAR, PH.D.**[1]

Practice Builder: With four college degrees in everything from business administration to psychology, and with experience ranging from marketing management to researching consumer behavior, you're known as a leading marketing theorist and practitioner. Would you explain your views on what the most important element in the successful marketing of a practice is?

Dr. Solar: *Differentiation*. It's one of the most basic principles of marketing. To be successful, a practitioner must closely identify markets, design services to fit patient needs, build on strengths and correct weaknesses, and, above all, be different in terms of services offered, promotion, or distribution or price of services. That's what is meant by the term "differentiation."

However, being different isn't enough. It's important to be different in ways that fit your patients' needs. In fact, differentiating yourself in meaningful ways is the most important strategy for professionals today.

PB: Why is it so important today when it never used to be?

Dr. Solar: A recent *Business Week* article addressed that very question. As *Business Week* pointed out, "Vast economic and social changes have made better marketing an imperative." As a people, we once shared homogeneous buying tastes and needs. But now the U.S. population has splintered into many different consumer groups, each with distinctive needs. As competition increases, consumers begin to look for services that more closely fit their personal needs.

Also, as everyone knows, there's growing competition in the professions. In fact, my analysis shows it will continue to increase beyond the year 1995. And among these practitioners, there will be plenty of savvy professionals who will be more than happy to please a more demanding public. Only the savvy will grow and prosper. Many others won't even survive.

PB: Could you show us how this growing sensitivity among professionals manifests itself?

Dr. Solar: Of course. There are plenty of examples: the physician who now comes to you for your convenience; the emergency center with long hours, lower costs than a hospital's, and no appointments required for regular care; obstetricians who cater to natural deliveries at home; all kinds of practitioners with special expertise in sports medicine; and now some practitioners even have Sunday hours for working families.

PB: How does a practitioner who's never planned this kind of marketing strategy before start?

Dr. Solar: The first step in differentiation is to select a group of patients to focus on. Be as specific as you can in describing your group—like senior citizens with incomes of $15,000 to $30,000 per year living in this particular small geographic area, or working mothers 25 to 45 years old, or members of a specific ethnic group within a 3-mile radius of your office.

Then find out what they want. Or you may decide to tell them what they need, in which case you'll still need to convince them that they should want it.

The next step is to *dare to be different*—to fill those needs. Here's a laundry list of ways to differentiate yourself. The professional should consider how each can be applied to his or her practice and also what's important to the prospective patient:

1. Image: Low, medium, or high style.

2. Office decor: It says a great deal about your quality and your prices.

3. Location: A professional building vs. a storefront vs. a mall or other choices. Take into account subway or bus line convenience if you target seniors or low-income patients and major road access and parking for the suburban patient. House calls? Mobile office?

4. Types of services: Specialization or full service, one-stop care from the generalist. An extra expertise that few provide or make known they provide.

5. Quality of service: Amount of time spent, effort expended, bedside manner, follow-up calls, patient education. Testimonials are very effective if permitted in your area.

6. Amount of service: Good, better, or best versions of your services provide more choices to fit specific needs at different prices.

7. Quality of training: Harvard, Yale, and Stanford still mean a lot. Board certifications do too *when* your prospective patients are educated about them. So tell them.

8. Staff training: How well your staff handles patients tells about you and the kind of physician you are.

9. Packaging: Putting two or more services and/or products together to make a complete program.

10. Timing: People want to be seen now, not in 3 weeks.

11. Availability: At their convenience, perhaps early morning, late afternoons, early evenings, or weekends.

12. Payment options: Cash, billing, installment terms, credit cards, electronic funds transfer (*EFT*) where monthly or quarterly installment payments are automatically deducted from the patient's checking account.

13. Pricing: High, medium, or low. Loss-leader pricing, discounts for cash payment, or discounts to members of certain groups or clubs. Early bird discounts for those who respond to an ad before its deadline, quantity discounts, or sliding scale discounts based on income. Be careful here. One shouldn't reduce one's pricing until all other avenues have been tried.

14. Samples: Free or nominal-charge consultations or screenings.

15. Special promotions. [See Chapter 11 for special ways to get your message out.]

PB: That's an extensive list. Obviously one physician wouldn't do all of them. How does he or she choose?

Dr. Solar: You choose what's important to your prospective clientele. You might not get it right the first or even second time, but if you think and talk about their needs, you'll hit the right combination sooner, rather than later. And when you do, you'll be all alone—at the top.

☐ HOW TO CULTIVATE THE IMAGE OF QUALITY

A California ophthalmologist differentiates himself from others performing radial keratotomy by pointing out that he has trained many practitioners in RK. So, he argues, if you're going to have RK, why go to a student when you can see the professor?

When J.M. opened his internal medicine practice in New Jersey last year, he publicized his education at Harvard. Are there practitioners with better credentials around? Certainly. But the ophthalmologist and internist differentiated themselves handsomely. And the reason comes down to *trust*.

In medicine, if prospective patients don't perceive that you're trustworthy, it's difficult to attract them. Even if you differentiate yourself in other ways, to make that message far more powerful, you should include reasons for people to entrust their care to you.

The Established Practitioner—For the physician who's been around awhile, a rich amount of background material exists from which to draw. No matter how bland a practitioner's resumé or curriculum vitae may look, there's plenty there—if you think about it from the patient's point of view. The following examples are distinctions that engender trust:

1. *Over X years' experience:* You must have at least 10 years behind you to use this platform. Anything less sounds lightweight. If you have more than 2 decades of experience, simply say "over 20 years' experience" to avoid being perceived as out-of-date. And what does your experience really mean? That there are things a physician can't learn in school. They only come with years of experience. All of this translates into trust.

2. *Honors and awards:* If you've been recognized by your peers or by third parties, tell people. But also tell them how difficult the competition was and how few professionals receive these honors. If it wasn't difficult, mention the requirements you had to meet to win. That's impressive enough.

3. *Published articles or books:* When you're in print, you're automatically an expert. So inform patients and prospects about your book, your chapter in a book, or your articles in *The Jordanian Journal of Back Care*. No publications? Consider publishing your own booklets. With desktop publishing these days, it's easy. Then you'll be an expert.

4. *Achievements:* Diplomate or fellow status is not impressive by itself because few people know what it means. So you must tell people that it took 3 years of study and passing a difficult examination that only 49% of professionals pass the first time they take it. Now such status becomes impressive and creates trust.

5. *Number of patients:* If you've seen a particular case often, prospective patients feel more comfortable about your ability to deal with it. After all, how many back, stomach, or throat problems do you have to diagnose before you get it down pat. So the distinction of having helped hundreds or thousands of people with similar problems is a strong one.

6. *Memberships:* When a patient was recently asked why he chose

a particular allergist, he said because when he looked in the *Yellow Pages*, that practitioner had more letters after his name than any of the others. They were all memberships. The fact that you pay multiple dues appears to be impressive.

The Young Practitioner—Physicians just starting out may believe they have nothing to differentiate themselves that would help them establish trust. Wrong. Below you'll discover a list of ways that effectively accomplish that task.

1. *Testimonials:* In any endeavor, these are powerful promoters. But pick testifiers who have a lot of respect in your community. If not, use an "average" patient with whom prospective patients can identify. (Check state regulations for guidelines.)

2. *Your greatest case story:* By describing your greatest case, people know that you might accomplish the same for them. Your impressive story creates trust.

3. *Continuing education:* You can make the case that you not only keep up with the latest developments, but you surpass legal requirements for continuing education hours. You have spent x hours in the last 2 years alone. And you do this because of your commitment to bring your patients the latest techniques. Therefore, by implication, if patients are interested in breakthrough knowledge, you're the one to see.

4. Community service: If you do work for the school system or volunteer for a nonprofit group, make people aware of it. Prospective patients tend to trust practitioners with a good heart.

5. Personal standards: Explaining your personal standards underscores your unwavering commitment to excellence. You've made a commitment to the best care for your patients.

How to Get the Word Out—After you've picked a strategy for differentiation, the question becomes which avenues of communication to use. First, inform your existing patient base to keep patients coming and to help boost referrals. Everyone likes to refer to an expert they trust.

Share this information in your quarterly mailings or newsletter. Incorporate the information into your practice brochure. Also share information with any "leave-behinds" you have for audiences at your speeches or seminars.

For external promotion, place your trust-producing prose in the *Yellow Pages*. It's a battleground where you must significantly differentiate yourself or lose the war. If you advertise in newspapers or other media, the message should appear there. Direct mail is another fine medium for these strategies. Here you have the added advantage of unlimited space in which to wax poetic and be convincing.

And the effect of all this? Those who don't know you will respect you before they come through the door. And those who do know you will respect you even more.

☐ COMPETITIVE INTELLIGENCE FOR THE INTELLIGENT COMPETITOR

"I know I need to differentiate my practice from those of my colleagues, but how do I do that?" questioned Florida orthopedic surgeon R.S. Inasmuch as R.S. was a new practitioner in town, it was a crucial question. Here's what he did.

Competitive Analysis—R.S. needed to understand that to differentiate, he first needed to analyze the existing competition. Without this all-important information, chances are he would have ended up as an indistinguishable look-alike with no competitive advantage—a fatal first step for a new entry in a hotly competitive market.

First, he made a list of his direct competitors—other orthopedic surgeons within 5 miles of his office. Then he made a list of other competitors—nearby general practitioners, sports medicine specialists, podiatrists, and chiropractors.

Next, he determined the characteristics most important in each of the competing practices and listed them as follows:

1. Target patients: demographics of the primary patients each competitor wanted to attract
2. Kind of services they provide
3. Education and expertise: overall and specifically competitive specialties
4. Experience: years in practice; years in present location
5. Patient contact: are aides used extensively to give the feeling of impersonal service, or do your competitors give highly personal service?
6. Pricing: low, medium, or high
7. Image: a judgment call about the quality of the practice from the patients' viewpoint
8. Hours of availability
9. Convenience of location
10. Quality of equipment: what kind, how modern?
11. Practice promotion: public relations, advertising, and the media used

12. Promotional claims
13. Approximate promotional budget

Intelligence Gathering—R.S. used the above characteristics as headings and then came up with the information for each competitor. Some information was easily gathered from the *Yellow Pages*, newspapers, and by requesting a practice brochure. From the promotion material, he understood their claims. From the media they used for ads and the frequency of the advertising, he estimated their promotional budgets.

For the remaining information he had a staff member call and ask for pricing, services, equipment, and so forth. He even had a staff member visit his main competitor as a patient. In addition, suppliers and former patients of those competitors proved invaluable sources of information. His sheets filled quickly.

Strengths and Weaknesses—To understand exactly how to compete, R.S. realized he needed a more structured analysis of his data. For this, he used a one-dimensional marketing research grid to compare each variable. All competitors (including himself) were assigned a number to identify them, and then each was positioned on a continuum depending on how well they performed in each category. R.S. is the practice identified as no. 1 (Fig 3–1).

Clear Understanding—Having thus illustrated these and other characteristics, R.S. reached his conclusions. He realized that his state-of-the-art equipment and relatively low pricing were points of differentiation. Comparisons led him to make some changes.

First, he realized he was underpriced for the area. So he raised his prices to equal those of the no. 4 practice, except for initial exams and office visits, which he kept low. Next, he decided to outspend his competitors in promotional dollars. If done well, this would win him a much larger market share immediately. And he would emphasize breakthroughs in orthopedics in his promotion and how he was the *only* practice in the area with such advanced equipment.

Results—The pricing changes alone increased the practice gross by 17%. With the tripling of his promotional budget to $2,100 per month, after 3 months' time the practice gross jumped an average $14,200 per month or 6.8 times return on promotional dollars invested.

"Without really understanding what my colleagues were doing, I couldn't figure out what I should be doing. . . . My price hike and my expanded promotions came straight out of that competitive analysis."

Experience:		
1 4 3		2
Low	Medium	High
Modern Equipment:		
4 3 2		1
Low	Medium	High
Pricing:		
1 4	2 3	
Low	Medium	High
Amount of Promotion:		
2 1	4 3	
Low	Medium	High

FIG 3–1.

☐ Market Research From the *Yellow Pages*

The *Yellow Pages* directory stands as a fountain of research about your competition. For instance, use it to identify how many competitors you really have in your area, to determine new competitors moving in, and to find out the marketing message of each. By the quality of their ads, you'll also be able to find out how sophisticated your competitors' marketing strategies have become and whether your competitors are more of a threat now than they were a year ago.

Read the book each year to keep your finger on the pulse of your market.

☐ USING PRICING AS A MARKETING STRATEGY

Historically, physician S.R.'s busyness became unbusy during the last 2 ½ weeks of each year. He usually took a vacation then, but for personal reasons last year he couldn't. The prospect that faced him: To sit in his office for 2 ½ weeks feeding the fish. But he wasn't the type to sit.

Instead, S.R. sent a mailing to all of his patients telling them of this usually slow time and how feeding the fish was so limiting. To avoid weeks of boredom, he would save his patients 20% of their medical bills if they came in during this slow period and rescued his fish from obesity. He also mentioned how they could save even more now because their deductibles are most likely paid. But if they waited until January, they'd face paying the deductible again.

It worked well. His solid middle-class patients liked the idea so much that many came in for minor problems they would have ordinarily ignored. In fact, he had one of his busiest 2 weeks of the year.

Strategy—Professionals, like other service industries, face great fluctuations in demand. But unlike businesses, most practitioners do little to smooth out the demand. Most give the staff vacation time; some feed the fish.

Many other service industries have found that different pricing structures during different times produce different demand levels. Examples: The movies cost $5 at night but $3 before 3 P.M. People have become used to the idea of paying different prices for the same service, knowing that the price is influenced by the time they acquire the service. Certainly people are more willing to pay this way than professionals have been willing to offer it, which is why S.R.'s experiment generated no negative comments from patients.

Results—Otorhinolaryngologist T.E. used the converse of this pricing strategy to generate more profitability. He raised his prices for the period of highest demand, namely emergencies. He added a 25% surcharge to all services delivered beyond normal office hours. His report: "I thought I might get some complaints, but no one balked. Everyone seemed to think it was reasonable to be charged more at 10:30 at night for my special trip."

☐ HALF OF A MARKETING PLAN FAILS

Podiatrist A.W. felt he needed to do something to build his practice and reverse the slow decline he'd experienced during the last 18 months. After surveying how other practitioners were expanding, he decided he needed to purchase a laser. Not that he believed he really needed one to provide better service. But it would work as a marketing tool.

After $30,000 of expense, the downward trend was unchanged even though he'd announced the new equipment in his newsletter. What went wrong?

Half of a Marketing Plan—A.W. was right. Today, a laser can make a practice appear progressive, innovative, and on the cutting edge. But it will have an impact only if lots of new prospective patients are told of the development with exciting verbiage. Certainly spending $30,000 should make any practitioner excited. Notifying existing patients in a low-key, bland newsletter isn't sufficient to get a solid return on $30,000. So outreach into the community is a must. After thinking over how to achieve a complete marketing plan, he had an ad and a flyer created similar to the ad shown in Figure 3–2 that focused on laser technology and what it offers. The marketing strategy was now complete.

Conclusion—Half a marketing strategy doesn't generate profits, only losses. So remember to consider all important variables of the plan.

☐ LOCATING MULTIPLE OFFICES BY MEDIA COVERAGE

The newspaper campaign for Northeast plastic surgeon M.S. was producing big returns: 27 calls per week yielding 6.1 cases. Over 80% of these patients lived near his office even though his ad covered the entire metropolitan area. He reasoned that he would get more re-

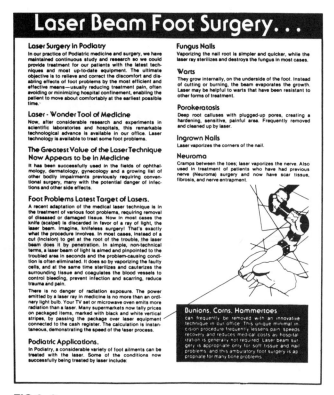

FIG 3–2.

Revving Up From a Cold Start

Can anything be more difficult in today's competitive environment than opening a practice cold? "Lots of things," says R.B., a family practitioner who opened "cold" 6 months ago. With intelligence and a personality to match, she methodically chose a site, launched the office, and within 30 days collected $8,000. Not a bad first month.

Making Contacts—Much of the groundwork to produce patient flow was laid prior to her opening. R.B. recognized that she had to meet people and make contacts. Lots of them. Her goal: to have 1,000 contacts open their doors to her *before* she opened her doors to them.

Going door–to–door, R.B. surveyed homes between 4:30 and 8:30 P.M. and on Saturdays. She asked questions so people were willing to talk with her and give her their opinions. Her introduction: "Good afternoon. I'm Dr. B_____, and I'm new in the area. I'm considering opening up a family practice in this community. If you have a moment, I'd like to ask you a few questions about your community." She went on to ask if they liked the area, how long they had lived there, if they thought it would be a good area in which to open an office, and if they could recommend a good place to live.

Surveys like this are tantalizing door-openers. An easy way to involve prospects and put them at ease. Time spent per person: 5 minutes. Time required to canvass the area: 6 weeks.

During the survey, R.B. jotted down the contacts' names and addresses, plus any small personal items of note. Each night she personalized a preprinted note, thanking those she'd seen that day for their input. And that she'd let them know the outcome of her survey in which they'd helped so much. The envelopes were hand addressed.

But did it work? Terrifically! Her first ten patients came directly from her survey work. And not only that, they turned out to be excellent referrers, accounting for her first 15 referrals.

Here's how she cultivated them. Three days prior to opening, R.B. sent a letter announcing her office opening. In it, she thanked the contacts again for their participation and reiterated how valuable their input was in helping select their community. She also included a separate sheet about her qualifications plus a special "thank you" coupon good for a discount.

Three months later, R.B. sent another letter. The thrust: "I'm doing so well in practice thanks to your input . . . thanks again . . . please call me if I can help, since it would be a privilege to care for you. . . . " And she sent additional follow-up in the form of quarterly newsletters and holiday greetings. These repetitive messages cultivated prospects and made the system work.

To assure a quick, positive cash flow, she added newspaper advertising to the promotional mix. Running twice a week, the 3-column × 6-in. ad started fast and continues to pull well today at the 6-month mark.

The ad's copy strategy introduces "the new doctor in town." In it, the copy explains R.B.'s background and qualifications. And by implication, that people receive more up-to-date techniques from her than from established practitioners. The ad's results the first month alone: 20 new patients.

"I'd worked in offices before starting my own practice, so I'd seen how haphazard practice building has been," R.B. explained. "Being extremely methodical was the *only* way I could have opened cold."

---

sponses if he had a second office serving another area that the same newspaper reached. After all, he was already paying $1,100 per week for the ad in that media.

When looking for a second location, he figured that the best place was the one with the least competition. In most cases this would be true. But not here.

Media Power—With media such as a major daily newspaper, you reach prospects far better than with far less effective weeklies, which are quickly "roundfiled." And with excellent promotion, your drawing area will expand far beyond your normal trading zone to the actual limits of the media coverage—if you have the locations to serve the prospects generated.

So the trick here is not to choose a secondary location by the competition factor only. First, make sure you're within the main coverage area of your winning media. Then check that the populace in the area has *similar demographics* to your original office. Why? Because some media do well with some people but not others. If you have a successful newspaper campaign, find another location to serve the other prospective patients that media are reaching. The results will be the same.

Then check the competition factor.

Weak Sisters?—If you've already got a second weak office and you're running a strong campaign, consider moving the second office to an area that will respond better to your promotion. Remember: A weak sister is weak for a reason. And dollars spent on a separate marketing effort for that office are much less productive than if spent in major media for the good of both or all offices.

Results—M.S. did open a second office 19 miles away to give him coverage in the newspaper's total market. The competition wasn't easy, but he was now able to draw from the entire two-county area reached by the paper. The new numbers: 46 calls per week yielding 10.3 cases total for the 2 offices. Comment: "I could never have gotten an office off the ground so quickly any other way. In fact, I would never have had a second office."

REFERENCE

1. Interview with D. L. Solar, Ph.D., Allergan Pharmaceuticals, 2525 Dupont Drive, Irvine, Calif.

■ CHAPTER 4
Time And Money: How Much You'll Need Of Each

☐ EVERY PRACTITIONER'S FIRST MAJOR HURDLE

As seen in the discussion on the one-page marketing plan, the budget you assign to your promotions is an important step. According to a well-respected economist, it can be the all-important step. According to Dr. Duran Bell,[1] a University of California professor, when making the decision to promote your practice, a professional's first major hurdle is not which market to target or what strategy to employ. It's deciding to spend resources.

"Building a practice takes work, thinking, and money. These are the investments of time, energy, and cash. Of course, there are numerous ways to promote practices, and each way has a different cost. But the point is that in one way or another, they all cost."

A Different Environment—Dr. Bell notes that in previous years, the economic factors were 180° different than they are today. Then, there was little incentive to invest in practice building. But in every profession including medicine, there is now an oversupply of practitioners, a demand that is not keeping pace with supply and increasing competition.

"In competitive arenas, owners must plow back resources into development. It's a must for survival. And it's this idea of investing to build a practice that is so foreign to most doctors," said Bell.

"No one ever had to do it before. Those who understand the importance of investing on an emotional level, as well as on an intellectual one, can act. They're the ones who'll win, because the majority of practitioners won't act—until it's too late."

☐ PROMOTIONAL BUDGETING FOR THE YEAR

Family practitioner L.M. called *The Practice Builder* advisory hotline recently to ask for suggestions on how to build his still young practice. During the conversation, the advisor asked what L.M.'s promotional budget was for the coming year. "Quite honestly," he answered, "I don't have one. Not that I don't have the money, just that I haven't set any aside."

L.M. isn't alone. Over 98% of the practitioners who call *The Practice Builder* advisory hotline have not set a promotional budget. And over 99% have not set specific practice goals. Without a budget and goals, these practitioners are driving a car at night without the lights on. They know the approximate direction they're headed, but can't really see where they're going.

Short and Sweet Budgeting—Specific goals come first: major growth of the practice/maintenance/a *turnaround* if the practice is in trouble. Quantify the goals, and then put your number in writing—for example, a 15% increase in gross, a 20% increase in patients.

Then set the budget. To set the ideal budget, first choose the strategy to accomplish the goal. Then figure the costs, see if you have enough in the bank to start up the campaign until cash flow takes over, and then put the final touches on reconciling the goals with the budget. *Remember: In a competitive environment, if you don't commit resources in either time or money, you'll never reach the goal.*

An Easier Way—Sometimes a rough estimate does just as well. Try these as guidelines for the medium-sized practice:

1. Use in-house, internal promotion or in-house public relations only: Dedicate 2% or 3% of *anticipated* gross for maintenance; 5% to 7% for moderate growth; 10% for major growth or a turnaround.

2. Use a public relations firm or advertising agency: Set aside 5% to 7% of anticipated gross for maintenance; 7% to 10% for moderate growth; and 10% to 15% for major growth or to heal a hemorrhaging practice. Beware of the biggest problem facing practitioners in this category: champagne goals on a beer budget.

Results—In L.M.'s case, his realistic goal for 1986 was a 10% increase in gross to a yearly total of $195,000. Not having done any prior internal promotion, and therefore having a lot of unharvested business, and being short of funds, he chose internal strategies to be executed in-house by him and his staff. Budget: 5% of anticipated gross or $9,750 per year or $812 per month.

"Setting the actual number helped give me the conviction to do something about my practice. Otherwise, it would be too easy to do nothing, just like last year."

☐ BIGGER BUDGETS, BIGGER PROFITS

A new *Practice Builder* study confirms for the professions what the advertising industry knew to be true for other businesses—that the bigger the promotion budget, the bigger the *percentage* of profits.

Increasing the average budget by five times boosts the number of new patients by four times. Since budgets tend to be small and the average expenditure from new patients during the first year with you are high (especially for surgeries), the leverage means big profits.

In other words, the *last dollars* you spend on promotion are *far more productive* than the first.

☐ HOW MUCH SHOULD I SPEND ON PRACTICE BUILDING?

Dr. Morton Walker[2] suggests there are at least four ways that professionals answer this frequently asked question:

1. The "I'll spend what I can afford" approach: This attitude treats promotion as an indulgence and reflects an underlying feeling that you're not serious about marketing your services. Subconsciously, you may be looking at marketing as a waste of time and money. A professional with this attitude should save his or her money and not promote at all.

2. The "I'll match the competition" approach: Because your colleague across the street runs a weekly 6-in. 2-column ad in the local shopper, your inclination might be to do the same. Fight the impulse. This is a defensive measure rather than a well-planned approach. It's better to make a careful analysis of your prospects and your goals, instead of blindly imitating the competition.

3. The "I'll invest a percentage of my gross income" approach: This forward-looking attitude makes two constructive assumptions: (a) Marketing is an investment for a larger future return; and (b) A concrete formula is needed to figure your budget allocation. The only danger with this attitude is that any allocation based on last year's figures might not be realistic for this year's promotional needs. Business cycles, after all, do fluctuate, and a downturn could leave you short of funds at a time when your promotional needs are greater than ever.

One physician we know figures 5.5% of gross annual income for promoting new business, no matter how much the economy fluctuates. Another method might be to spend 5% of your gross income for maintenance or slight business growth. Spend 10% for explosive growth or for maintenance during highly competitive periods.

4. The "I'll allocate so much per person" approach. Using this method, you take the number of new patients that entered your practice last year and designate a minimum value per head. Walker describes a veterinarian in the Midwest who assigns each new anticipated patient for the coming year $20 in budget money. He averages 1,000 office surgical operations a year on about 450 animals, his $9,000 annual budget helped him earn $188,000 in patient visits last year.

Another Tack—*The Practice Builder* recommends a fifth approach.

5. The "plan your goals and work your plan" approach. Take the time to write down exactly what you want to accomplish. Set numerical goals whenever possible—for example, 20% growth, $15,000 increase in gross profits, or 300 new patients. Then determine how many dollars the "average" new patient generates. A quick random check of your records and a little elementary math will yield this figure. Now decide how much you're willing to spend to gain that amount. Raise the sum for quicker growth, and lower it for maintenance.

There is, of course, a maximum. And that's the point where you are spending what each new patient brings in during his or her first series of visits with you. If you are spending to this break-even point, then you're still making a profit from referrals and repeat visits in the future. Most professionals will be conservative and spend considerably less. But that doesn't mean you can't spend up to your break-even point to build your base more quickly. Just be sure that you're attracting loyal, highly referring patients.

☐ PROMOTIONAL BUDGET DEPENDS ON PROFESSIONAL LIFE CYCLE

Just as people undergo life cycles, so do institutions, products, companies—and professional practices. Each of them experiences a birth, then a period of growth, followed by an era of maturity, which is ushered out with the onset of decline. Where your practice is positioned in its life cycle determines how much you need to spend on promotion.

If you're just starting out or first starting to promote, you need to spend substantially. In this birth phase, 10% to 20% of gross is not uncommon. The exact percentage is determined by how much growth you want and how high the marketing costs are in your area. Large cities cost the most; rural areas the least.

Establishing a Presence—The reason behind the large percentage is the need to establish an immediate recognition or presence in the marketplace. People don't respond the first or second time they see or hear your message. Rather, the average person takes five to seven repetitions before feeling comfortable enough to call for an appointment. And to gain these repetitions of the message, you must run your promotions often. Hence, the need for a large budget.

To achieve major growth during the growth phase also requires a large budget for the same reasons.

But if you're looking to maintain your practice that you've actively promoted during its earlier growth period and are now in the maturity phase, cut back moderately on the budget to about 5% or 10% of gross or even less. With your existing presence in the market, there's no need to overspend to maintain what you've built.

The Mature Practice—If you're looking to retire in the next few years, cut the promotional budget altogether and raise your fees. It's time to fully profit from the years you've invested in the practice by cutting the reinvestment that had been necessary for earlier expansion.

Competition also figures into the equation during the birth, growth, and maturity stages. The more there is, the more you'll need to spend.

☐ WHAT TO DO FIRST IN MARKETING?

Once you've analyzed your market, the competition, and your own practice, the question becomes where you should invest your promotional budget first. Here's the order that marketing consultant Paul Brosche[3] suggests for the best returns on a marketing dollar invested:

1. *Outdoor office signs:* If you have an opportunity for an outdoor sign, this comes first. For a one-time investment, your outdoor sign can continuously capture drive-by and pedestrian traffic, if it's well done. No other media can do so much for so long and so little (see Chapter 11).
2. *Recalls*: It's easier to continue selling a service to someone with whom you already have a relationship (see Chapter 6).
3. *Internal patient education:* It's easier to sell a new service to someone with whom you already have a relationship (see Chapter 6).

4. *Referrals*: Reinforce and reward all referrals, especially patients who are heavy referrers (see Chapter 7).

5. *Staff incentive programs:* The staff can recruit as well as you can, given the right incentives. And the programs don't cost anything unless they produce (see Chapter 7).

6. *Periodic internal promotion*: Brosche recommends sending letters to your existing patient base rather than using a less often read newsletter. Letters will keep up contact to protect your base from competitive raiders (see Chapter 8).

7. *Yellow Pages*: In no other medium are you likely to generate over $10 in receipts for every dollar invested. The volume of qualified prospects who use them makes the *Yellow Pages* a crucial buy (see Chapter 15).

8. *A balanced program of public relations and advertising or personal selling:* 66% of the average practice's gross comes from new dollars—people you haven't seen before. Public relations is limited in its ability to draw consistently, yet it adds great credibility to a practice. It also produces a synergistic effort when coupled with an ad program. Your personal selling can obviate or complement PR and advertising—but only *if* you pursue enough contacts *and* if you can sell. A dignified but effective advertising campaign is the choice for professionals who are uncomfortable with the idea of having to sell themselves (see Section III).

These are general guidelines for practices promoting largely to the public. They'll change in individual cases and for other other types of practices and are, of course, affected by the rest of your marketing plan.

☐ PLAN AHEAD

Anyone can sit down and dash off a promotion in an hour's time. But good promotion takes a goodly amount of time. Six to 8 weeks from conception to launch is a comfortable time to spend. Why so long? Because of the creative process.

As we've seen, you first need to delineate your target market, whether you're creating a promotional piece or advertising for the *Yellow Pages*, shoppers, direct mail, radio, or TV. That involves market research time. Then you must choose the right strategy—the big promise and all the little promises. More time. Then you write, you create. More time yet.

The Time Test—And here's the crucial point. Plan to put your creative writing aside for a few days so you can evaluate it with a fresh eye. What seemed award winning a few days before may now come across as tranquilizing. Using a fresh-eye process always produces better promotion. But it takes time.

Production also takes time. In direct mail, that's a week in art production, 1 to 2 weeks in printing, 3 to 7 days in the mailing house, and 3 to 10 days in the mail.

When do most mistakes occur? When rushing to meet a deadline. Better strategy: Plan ahead.

☐ RESPOND QUICKLY

This is an urgent reminder not to be caught in the same trap physician L.B. was. Last fall, he experienced a noticeable slowdown in his practice. When he actually studied the numbers, he should have called it a hemorrhage—a 20% drop from the previous year. But his overhead, of course, hadn't fallen 20%.

Even though he needed to market the practice, he hemmed and hawed into the new year. When he finally took the idea seriously, he discovered he couldn't produce and place promotion as quickly as he wanted or needed. In the meantime, the practice continued to

---

☐ The Three Secrets of Marketing

There are three secrets of marketing according to Jay Levinston in his book, *Guerrilla Marketing*.[4] Commitment. Investment. Consistency.

Commitment means if you don't generate positive results within 2 weeks, you don't throw in the towel. Without commitment, your marketing is impotent.

Investment means you commit enough time and/or money to achieve the goal. It means viewing it not as a cost of doing business, but as a conservative investment to make money. You invest in marketing the same way you invest in a blue-chip stock, which may retreat before it advances. Done well, marketing will contribute to slow, steady increases for you. And at the end of the year, you'll be able to say that you've invested $X and *earned* $X plus $Y in profits. That's just the way conservative investments are supposed to pay off.

Consistency means sticking with the media and messages you chose because those decisions were based on solid judgment. It also means not dropping from the public eye for long. For the public, your consistency means ever-increasing familiarity, which means growing confidence in you and income for you.

These three secrets are among the most valuable you can learn. And the most difficult to follow.

---

struggle, with less and less cash flow now available for the turnaround he so badly needed.

Plan Now—The idea is to be proactive and control your practice rather than playing the much more difficult, if not impossible, game of catch-up, or worse, becoming a passive victim of the market and growing competition.

Ask yourself—honestly—whether your image needs updating; whether a prospective patient looking at the practice might believe you're dated. Study your logo, stationery system, business card, and internal promotion. What do you see?

Plan Like a Business—If you're planning to promote at all in the next 12 months, now's the time to begin the process. Don't get caught in a time crunch. And avoid the procrastination that crippled L.B.'s efforts so badly.

☐ STRATEGY'S IMPORTANT BUT . . .

In marketing, strategy is mandatory, but execution is everything. A few years ago, doctors could ignore this maxim and get away with it. Today the competition is too stiff.

Ophthalmologist J.I. disliked the business aspects of his practice. When he decided to do a mailing to senior citizens, he oversaw the creative process but delegated the rest to his office manager.

Disastrous Results—What went wrong? Plenty. The mailing list the office ordered was for seniors within a 5-mile radius. The list received was for a city 25 miles away. But it didn't matter. The mailing finally went out 2 days before the deadline described in the material to receive a free cataract screening. The mailing was sent third class with a 5- to 15-day delivery time. Loss: $1,320.

To be successful, professionals must pay close attention to the grunt work—the hundreds of details that must be right to make marketing pay.

The best strategy in the world, for example, won't get you anywhere if a key mailing goes out incorrectly or if the copy to appear in your *Yellow Pages* ad is late. Today's marketplace is simply too sophisticated for anything but perfection.

Details, Details—Unfortunately, many practitioners think that the detail work is beneath them. They either delegate it to less skillful employees or ignore it altogether. The inevitable result: Their market share shrinks and *income declines*. Ironically, the practitioner blames the problem on the strategy.

Never view the grunt work in a begrudging way. Recognize that it is important that the envelopes are sorted correctly or that the newsletter is ready on time. If you don't focus on the details, you can be sure that a competitor will. Make it clear to employees that the route to the top is through excellence in execution. That requires painstaking attention to detail.

If you don't control your marketing function and aren't active in it, those with less to lose will lose more for you, not through malicious intent, but simply because they're not as smart as you are, and they don't think about those issues 27 hours a day. So of course, they'll produce less than you.

Supervision Needed—That means you can't delegate without very close supervision. You can't ask someone of lesser intelligence and with lesser vested interest to be responsible for the life-giving flow of the practice. To give up responsibility for bringing in new patients or continuing to attract existing patients is to start a slow suicide or at least to gamble on a greatly diminished health of the practice.

So you can delegate much of the work. Certainly do so, but supervise closely. What you can't delegate is the responsibility and involvement in the planning. For a prosperous practice, you know where the buck stops—and starts.

Professionals who focus on implementing as well as formulating strategies will enjoy sustained growth. The others may not be around to figure out what went wrong.

REFERENCES

1. Interview with Duran Bell, Ph.D., Professor of Economics, University of California, Irvine, Calif.
2. Walker M: *Advertising and Promoting the Professional Practice.* New York, Hawthorn Books Inc, 1979, p 54.
3. Interview with Paul Brosche, General Manager, The Practice Builder Ad Agency, Irvine, Calif.
4. Levinson J: *Guerrilla Marketing.* Boston, Houghton Mifflin Co, 1984, p 22.

■ PART 2   Your Tools

■ SECTION 1
New Ideas For Marketing And Promoting
Within: The Path Of Least Resistance And
Least Cost

■ CHAPTER 5
Projecting The Ultimate Image: Professional Vs. Retail; Effective Vs. Boring

☐ **PSYCHOLOGICAL FACTORS IN PATIENT RETENTION**

Patients stay with physicians who do three things for them—the physicians *understand* their problems; they *know* the solution, and they *care* about their patients. This is certainly easy enough to understand, but how do you translate these characteristics into action. How do you communicate your concern? Dr. Peter Fernandez,[1] noted practice consultant, offers concrete suggestions.

During the initial consultation, of course, you listen closely. Once you've got a handle on the patient's complaint, communicate it, perhaps by saying, "Let me see if I understand the situation." Then restate the problem, and after any discussion, comment, "Now I understand." These are simple words. But incredibly important ones, says Fernandez. Because patients don't leave a professional who understands them.

Involve the Patient—During the next phase, of course, you determine the course of treatment by conducting the physical exam, running tests, and examining records. The important thing is to talk the patient through it. Explain what your examination means so he'll know you know the right course. Involve patients, even exhaust them. The more obviously thorough you are, the more impressed they are.

The thoroughness of your examination has an ancillary benefit too. How thorough you are is directly related to the *number of referrals* patients make. Enthusiastic patients refer—merely satisfied ones don't.

At the end of the examination phase, look the patient directly in the eye and say, "I now know exactly what to do." The confidence you have in your own ability breeds the patient's confidence in you.

Accelerate Treatment—Then when recommending a course of treatment, remember: The more accelerated the treatment, the higher the percentage of patients who complete it. Studies show that when repeated treatments are needed, a schedule of three times per week generated 70% follow through. But treatments scheduled once a day had 90% completion, while those scheduled twice a day hit 95%. Compression conveys a sense of urgency. The same principle is true for all specialties.

☐ SHOW YOU CARE

Having shown that you understand a patient and know the best course of treatment, the third critical characteristic is to demonstrate that you care. The following are 17 different ways to show you care. Remember: Talk is cheap, but your actions prove the point.

1. *Be available.* Give every patient your business card with your private office and home numbers. You're in the busijness of providing health care. If you don't want to be available to your patients, you should be in manufacturing.
2. *Recognize every patient.* When someone places himself or herself in a physician's hands, it's unnerving not to be recognized.
3. *Offer extended hours.* Do you want your employees taking time for personal appointments between 9 A.M. and 5 P.M.? Other employers don't either.
4. *Hire a hostess*—not a receptionist. A positive, bubbly person who loves everyone should greet all comers. Keep the crusty grumps in the back office and off the phones.
5. *Recapture no-shows.* Contact those who miss or cancel their appointments. It not only shows you care, it makes you income. One no-show per day costs you $10,000 per year. Three cost you $30,000.
6. *Keep a social profile* on every patient. Then ask about their golf, fishing, or grandchild. Don't talk about yourself.
7. *Make your patients feel needed,* wanted, appreciated, and important. One way: Ask them for a favor.
8. *Look them in the eye.* This is the single most important activity a practitioner can do to build trust.
9. *Touch them.* On the shoulder, on the hand.

☐ **Thank You, Thank You**

Because making patients feel important is a key to retention, California physician R.M. found a way to create that bond. Once a year he writes a letter to each of his patients thanking them for allowing him to be their practitioner and inviting them back when they need him again. He finds that this personal and unexpected attention improves his relations and creates a loyalty he can measure in numbers. Since he started his thank you letters 2 years ago, patients transferring to other practitioners have dropped off, plus visits by past patients are up over 25% from 2 years before.

10. *Concentrate only on them.* When with a patient, be with that patient. Remove all else from your mind. This is the essence of quality time.

11. *Lift their spirits.* Give hope. But avoid jokes. Why? Because the patient will waste your time by telling you one in return. Certainly avoid off-color jokes, even with hard hats. This is the surest way to stop them from referring their mothers, wives, and other women.

12. *Slow down* when you're running behind. When pressured, force yourself to slow down to avoid a frenzied appearance and making patients feel cheated. You'll also get more done in less time without mistakes.

13. *Inform as you perform.* Tell them your game plan. It makes people feel more in control as well as respected.

14. *Show and tell.* Visuals increase understanding—models, charts, illustrations, computer graphics. They make people feel more comfortable.

15. *Explain the function* of each piece of equipment and every diagnostic tool as you use it.

16. *Insist on patient convenience.* Eliminate waiting time. Make sure that nothing in your practice rubs your patients the wrong way.

17. *Give.* This is a winning attitude in any service profession. The more you give, the more you get back.

☐ **THE SPECIAL TOUCHES THAT REALLY COUNT**

If those behaviors and attitudes will set you apart from the competition, similar small touches can also make quite a difference. The following is a list of special touches—small acts that put you in the best light and are remembered totally out of proportion to the effort behind them.

1. *Flowers*: Red carnations on Valentine's Day, green ones on St. Patrick's, and so on. Most male practitioners forget how wonderful a flower can make a woman feel.

2. *New patient bulletin board*: People love to see their names in print. A message board that welcomes and thanks patients by name fills this basic need for recognition.

3. *Testimonial display*: While they're waiting, have your patients fill out a sheet explaining how they've been helped or not helped by you. Have a box to check if they would like the sheet posted on your "thank you" board. If permission is granted, post the testimonial. You receive positive feedback that can be displayed and negative comments to alert you to problems that need correcting. And your patients gain recognition on the board. For a permanent record, cycle older testimonials into a waiting room album.

4. *Birthday cards*: Everyone sends holiday cards so there's nothing special there. Instead, send cards on other occasions, especially the patient's birthday. It's a touch everyone will remember.

5. *Personal file*: Have a place in your patients' files to make notes about their personal interests, spouses' work, children's activities, business interests, vacations, and hobbies. During the next visit, ask about one or more of those areas. Personal concern in an impersonal world is not easily forgotten.

6. *Follow-ups*: Mail a personal letter after a new patient's first visit, thanking each one for the faith placed in you and assuring the person that you will justify that faith. After the last visit in a series or when the next visit is months away, send a personal letter thanking the person for the trust, and state that you're looking forward to helping him or her in the future. The first letter surprises and pleases the patient. The second one astonishes them.

7. *Lasting bond*: Recently, a patient canceled a checkup appointment due to a death in his family. The physician sent a plant from a

---

☐ The Ultimate in Bedside Manner

Physicians naturally make follow-up calls to patients after treatment. But to provide the ultimate in care, and to create the ultimate in loyalty, do what internist T.T. does.

Whenever T.T. refers patients to other specialists, she follows up directly with the patients to make sure they're satisfied with the referral and the care they're receiving. "This way I have ongoing feedback about the specialists I refer to. And, of course, the patients are absolutely flabbergasted that the nontreating physician would care about them. This one activity creates real devotion."

---

florist—not cut flowers that would be gone in a week but a potted plant to remind the patient of the doctor's kindness for years to come. The patient will never change practitioners. On life's extraordinary occasions, send a lasting gift.

☐ THE MAKING OF AN EXPERT

Psychiatrist D.T. called *The Practice Builder* advisory hotline to ask, "How do I get more major corporations to refer their employees to me?" After probing his background, we found his recent research on stress had application for increased productivity in the workplace. Recommended strategy: Position him as an expert in work-related stress to encourage corporate referrals.

Translation—First, recast the stress research from academic into business terms, highlighting those sections of interest to personnel managers, employee assistance program (EAP) directors, and the like. To grab attention, headline the research with the most unusual finding. Develop a list of large businesses in the area and use direct mail to reach them. Follow up with phone calls to them to ask for referrals.

Also, develop a list of appropriate media (newspapers, magazines, radio, and TV) that reach these key business people. Send the media a press release outlining the most newsworthy of the findings. Again, follow up by phoning the editors and reporters one week after the mailing. If you are presented as an authority in the media, you're seen as one in the eyes of the public.

Results—Four newspaper articles and two radio shows. Even though some were broadcast at times with small audiences or in poorly read media, this was far from discouraging. Why? Because after each appearance or publication, D.T. sent letters and reprints to his prospect list of personnel managers and to the remaining media. The tag "expert" was now applied more freely. The aura was forming.

More Research—The next step was to develop another piece of research—a new stress survey. D.T. made his findings available to companies and to the same media. This time, not only did D.T. receive more media exposure and increased employee referrals from corporations, he also received an unexpected bonus—a large consulting contract from a Fortune 500 company.

"I learned two big things from this—first, to rewrite the material important to my specific audience to make it even more interesting for them; and second, once the media picks up on it, to leverage it by announcing the article or appearance to others and keep the ball rolling. My caseload is up, and the spin-offs really sweeten the payoff."

☐ WRITE FOR CREDIBILITY

Even though he didn't expect to make any money or even get published, Dr. T.W. wrote a book. Actually at 32 pages, it's more appropriate to call it a booklet. But this treatment plan for headaches has been his best practice builder ever.

Strategy: Talk is not only cheap, but it's often forgotten moments later. But when you're in print, you're memorable. And you've also become an expert. So T.W. self-published his plan and publicized it.

"Originally I wrote it because I had it in me and I figured I could help some people. But as word-of-mouth about the booklet grew, requests grew and so did appointments. I decided then that I'd help the word-of-mouth along by advertising it."

He ran two 5×7-in. ads per week in his local newspaper. The ads offered a free copy of his booklet just for dropping by or calling in. Smartly, he gave two ways to respond.

Results: In the first 30 days, he gave out 117 copies. He also booked 29 new patients. Most will spend in excess of $500 each with him.

"Now I'm busier and these highly motivated patients have an incredible respect for me *before* they even come in."

For a nationwide list of book printers that can produce 10 to 10,000 copies of a book, catalog, or a booklet, order a copy of *The Directory of Short-Run Book Printers* from Ad-Lib Publications (P.O. Box 1102, Fairfield, IA 52556-1102).

☐ HOW TO STOP LOSING BUSINESS

A New Hampshire GP was befuddled. In the last 6 months, the number of files to be transferred to other practitioners doubled. Was it increased competition? His new pricing? Some other problem in the practice? How could he identify the problem and stop the hemorrhage?

The Exit Survey—He smartly adapted an idea from the personnel field. When an employee leaves, most astute corporate personnel departments hold an exit interview to learn what went wrong so they can better retain their employees in the future. The GP did the same thing, but with his patients.

"When a patient requested his or her chart be transferred, we separately sent the person a one-page questionnaire together with a postage-paid envelope addressed to the office."

"We made sure the patient understood that answers were to be anonymous. Then we asked him or her to rate our services to help improve them. We used a rating scale from one for poor to five for great and asked the patient to rate our waiting time, ability, concern shown, pricing, covenient office hours, and so on. Then we asked the open-ended question of why the patient left the practice."

Results—"From a few of the returned questions, we found price was one problem. That was not surprising, since I'd just raised them. But I also discovered my new front desk employee was cold and sometimes downright nasty. I'd had no idea."

The practitioner also learned about a new competitor who was sending out direct mail. "One patient actually sent me a sample of the mailer. Even I admitted it was great. But at least, now I knew the problems so I could figure out what to do."

☐ MARKETING YOUR CREDENTIALS

Two questions: First, what's the first thing a patient does when he or she sits down in your reception room? Answer: Grab something to read. Second question: How much does your patient know about you and your professional qualifications? Answer: Probably very little or nothing.

Voilà. That's the perfect opportunity to expand your internal marketing program. Strengthen patient confidence in your professional abilities. And provide material for patients to share with their family and friends who may need your services.

The Reception Room Resume—It's *brief* (three or four short paragraphs), *professional* (focusing on honors; association and society memberships; service on boards, committees; speeches and publications), and *personal* (translating everything into patient-oriented benefits).

Starting point: Probably to update your practice brochure biography, expanding it to include recent professional activities and their significance to your reader.

If you find yourself resisting this personal promotion, remember that every year you take hundreds of hours of accredited continuing education courses. You attend lectures, seminars, and professional association and society meetings. You participate in study groups and even serve on committees and task forces.

It's all done to improve your skills, increase your knowledge, and better serve your patients. So don't be shy about publicizing your efforts, but do it in ways that are meaningful to your patients.

Results—Otolaryngologist J.H. thought he'd tell his patients a little about himself. So he printed up his curriculum vitae and put several in plastic sleeves around the waiting room. Patient comments: "I had no idea it took so much training to become an ENT specialist." "I sure feel that I'm in good hands." One man said, "I didn't know you were that smart!"

Your resumé or curriculum vitae is nothing more than a *marketing tool*. It is not simply a fact sheet blandly stating your background, but should be a carefully crafted promotion. In fact, it's far more convincing because its format is so uncommercial. Given the fact that 99.9% of doctors don't view their CV or resumé this way, when a patient reads one, he or she is bound to be impressed.

Take a look at your own background. With a few colorful words to adequately describe it and a professional presentation of the information, you too can be seen as *the* well-qualified physician in your area. And the addition to the bottom line? More referrals and better retention.

☐ HOW TO CREATE THE IMAGE OF AN EXPERT AND AVOID LOOKING DATED

Iowa physician L.C. began to notice a long-term slide for the first time in over 25 years of practice. In studying what was happening, he uncovered the fact that his long-time patients were staying with him, but he couldn't seem to keep younger people. Few came, and of those who did, few stayed.

L.C. then did the smart thing just as that New Hampshire GP had done. To those who hadn't been back in 2 or more years, L.C. sent out a confidential survey to which the patient could respond anonymously. The purpose: To find out why they weren't coming back. His surprising discovery: The former patients told him he wasn't up-to-date.

The Perception vs. the Reality—L.C. was shocked. He knew he kept on top of medical advances and consistently delivered good, up-to-date treatment. Admittedly his practice wasn't the Mayo Clinic, but it wasn't chopped liver either.

The marketing consultant L.C. called was quick to point out the reason for the survey results. When the consultant walked into the practice, he *felt* he was entering an old practice. The place looked drab. The furniture was clean and functional, but dated. The outdoor sign was dated. The decorating appointments looked 1960-ish, not timeless. And the office was sparse.

No wonder people in their 30s and younger didn't respond. L.C. may have provided up-to-date care, but people perceived the practice as old even before they saw him.

The Strategy—Two key concepts needed to be put into operation here. First, no one leaves an expert. If patients perceived L.C. as the best around, there'd be no problem with recalls or referrals. But they were prejudiced at the start. And the consequence was diminished credibility. Second, no one can be an expert if they're not perceived as state-of-the-art. This is self-evident.

Here's what the marketing consultant advised. His question: What's the first thing you do when you're about to put your house up for sale? You paint it. Do the same thing for a practice. It's amazing what a fresh coat of paint can do for the spirit. And the consultant suggested that L.C. have the free-standing building painted a more modern color than the earth tones and dull browns of the 1970s. The choice: bright white with teal green awnings and small accents of ice blue and creamy burgundy. Also added: a bright white picket fence for a timeless touch. The right highlights in modern-looking colors solidly positioned L.C. as a practitioner of today.

Other Touches—Then came a new sign. Also in a teal green background with bright white letters and lighted from within, the sign reinforced the new image. So did the copy: "Today's Family Medicine." L.C.'s name and phone number were shown below.

Then the inside of the office was also painted, but in subdued pastel versions of the color scheme. The waiting room furniture was replaced. And the magazine mix was redone to cater to a wider age range of tastes and interests.

The nurses and assistants received more modern-looking garb. And each received a practice patch for their uniforms. The patch carried the practice's new logo and positioning tag line, "Today's Family Medicine," in the new practice colors.

And More Credibility—The consultant noticed that even though L.C. had a rich background, no patient would ever know about it. True, a few plaques dotted the exam rooms, but the consultant judged the number too few and the impression too limp to generate an "oh, wow" response.

So he took all the plaques, awards, honors, and commendations and concentrated them in the waiting room. He was careful *not* to use those over 15 years old. Instead, he framed or plaqued the newer ones that had been boxed and put away. How many honors, awards, and papers that would be impressive to patients did he put on the walls? Twenty-two. And when he got them up, he actually went back and added four more. Now every patient was sure L.C. was an up-to-date expert. They could read the writing on the wall.

By the way, all the assistants also had their plaques hung on a separate wall. So not only was L.C. an expert, everyone in his office was, too.

More Promotion—The new face-lift was carried over into other areas. The business cards and stationery system now reflected the new tag line and colors. And a *Yellow Pages* ad was added to extend the themes and start bringing in new younger patients now that he could keep them.

Concept: Work within the practice first and correct all the problems there before promoting outside. Bringing in a substantial number of new patients before the practice is finely honed will only damage your reputation. In large markets, it can hurt. In smaller ones, it can kill.

Results—The program worked. Within 6 months after the changes, referrals were up 18% over the year before and climbing. A spectrum of patient ages was starting to come back with more younger families who now felt confident in the practice. L.C.'s summary: "I always thought you just had to practice the best medicine you could and everything would take care of itself. Well, I was wrong. This taught me I also needed to communicate who I am in different ways than I would usually think of communication—signs and furniture, even wall decorations. It makes sense now, but I must admit I only realized this in hindsight."

☐ THE RULE OF 225

New research[2] defines exactly how much patient dissatisfaction actually can cost your practice. Of patients with billings of $100 or more

- 84% remained loyal to the practice if the complaint was solved quickly;
- 54% remained loyal if the complaint was resolved—even if it took some time;

- Only 19% remained with the practice after complaining when the problem wasn't resolved;
- 9% remained loyal after identifying a problem but not complaining about it.

That first figure again underlines the importance of listening and communicating thoroughly with disgruntled patients. And treating them with the utmost respect as if they're the most important people in the world to you—because they are.

But other experts have looked beyond the office itself and suggest that the impact continues even after the dissatisfied patient leaves your office. Public relations pros like Scott Montgomery[3] of Salvati, Montgomery & Sakoda in Costa Mesa, Calif. believe there's a bigger reason to be concerned about the impact of unhappy patients. "On the average, when anyone dissatisfied leaves your practice," says Montgomery, "that person will tell 15 people how awful, uncaring, and unprofessional you are, no matter how untrue. And because of the way bad news travels, each of those 15 people turn around, and each tell another 15 people. That's a grand total of 225 people who would rather go to anyone other than you."

Unfortunately, Montgomery notes that good news works only by the "Rule of Five." A good recommendation reaches two people who each tell only two other people.

☐ HOW TO DEAL WITH AN ANGRY PATIENT

Every practice has an angry patient every once in awhile. Someone calls or comes in irate with the practice or the practitioner. The first step in controlling the damage is to keep the anger from spreading. When someone comes in seething, remove the person from the waiting room into a private room. Then handle the walk-in or the call the same way with these three steps[4]:

1. Do not disturb the patient's release of emotion. Allow him or her to vent all the anger without any interruption. Any effort to intervene will only incur resentment and more anger.

2. Even if you know where the patient's remarks are headed, do not anticipate his or her comments. People want to feel that they are understood and taken seriously. Let the patient fully express his or her anger in the individual's own way and own words.

3. After you've given the person an opportunity to fully describe their problem, respond. When you do speak, lower your voice, breathe easily, and reduce your rate of speech. Say neutral comments such

☐ Waiting Room Fever

When your waiting room backs up, you've got lots of ruffled feathers to smooth out. So if a patient waits more than 30 minutes to see you, reduce your fee a small but noticeable amount. And explain the reason for the reduction—that their time is also valuable.

They'll remember your thoughtfulness, not their earlier irritation.

---

as "I'd like to help you." Then use the "three Fs"—Feel, Felt, Found. That means: "I know how you feel. I've felt that way myself. I've found that this may help." Never argue. Always agree that their feelings are justified. But perhaps their facts are not complete.

Introduce these steps during a staff meeting. Have everyone practice once or twice. And then you'll be ready for the inevitable.

Properly handling complaints can build patient loyalty. And remember: The reverse is also true.

☐ HOW BEING BUSY CAN HURT YOUR BUSINESS

Too many of today's physicians have created the image that they are too busy to provide proper care. As they scurry from room to room, glacing at a chart and only stopping for curt conversations, these professionals are unwittingly creating a damaging impression in their patients' minds: They're too harried to provide the kind of care the patients want to get in return for their hard-earned dollars.

The pressures of the modern practice may cause a professional to push to accomplish more in less time, but the cost is often an insidious erosion of patient confidence and then a loss of those patients.

The simple solution: Sit down. By sitting down each time you see a patient, you create an impression of spending time and feeling concern. Chances are that you'll spend about as much time with the person as you would when you remain standing ready to rush off. Your patients will appreciate the increased attention and be more likely to stay in your care.

Denver physician P.E. changed his work behavior and now makes it a point to sit down with each patient. "I now see more patients than I ever did before," he says. "But I act and feel more relaxed. And my patients sense it, too. Because I sit down with each of them, they feel that they're getting their money's worth."

REFERENCES

1. Interview with Peter Fernandez, D.C., Practice Motivation International, 10812 Gandy Boulevard North, St Petersburg, FL 33702.
2. Arlene Malech, Technical Assistance Research Project, cited in "Increasing credibility in communications." *Communication Briefings*, August 1986, p 3 (P.O. Box 587, Glassboro, NJ 08028).
3. Interview with Scott Montgomery, Salvati, Montgomery & Sakoda, Costa Mesa, Calif.
4. Decker B: Defusing anger. *Decker Communication Report*, July 1986, p 2 (607 N Sherman Ave, Madison, WI 53704).

■ CHAPTER 6
Easily Keeping Patients; Easily Boosting Recalls

☐ HOW TO FIND OUT IF YOUR INTERNAL PROMOTION WORKS

There's a marketing adage that warns, "strategy's important, but execution's everything." To find out if his internal promotion was achieving what he hoped, Minnesota physician T.S. used a tool we glanced at in Chapter 5. T.S. developed a survey that he mailed to all of the patients he'd seen in the last 3 years.

The survey was sent bulk rate. The cover letter was written on practice stationery, sent in an office envelope, metered to look business-like. The cover letter asked the patient to do T.S. a personal favor and take 60 seconds to fill out the enclosed questionnaire. It also asked that they not include their name to assure confidentiality. A postage-paid envelope was enclosed for a no-cost response.

How Are We Doing?—The questionnaire asked the patient to rank aspects of the practice along a continuum of poor, needs some improvement, average or acceptable, above average, exceptional. Here were the questions asked:

- Are our phones answered promptly?
- Is the staff courteous and helpful on the phone?
- Can you get an appointment as quickly as you want?
- Are our hours convenient for you?
- Is there enough easy parking at our office?
- Is the length of time spent in our waiting room acceptable?
- Is our front desk helpful, friendly, and fast? (If not, please indicate who was not. Your confidentiality is assured.)

- Are our other assistants helpful, friendly, and fast? (If not, please indicate who was not. Your confidentiality is assured.)
- Does the doctor take enough time with you?
- Does the doctor give you enough personal attention and concern?
- Does the doctor involve you enough in decisions?
- Does the doctor explain recommendations and other information clearly?
- If you have ever had an emergency, did we respond as expected?
- Does the office keep you sufficiently informed about medical advances and other items of importance?
- Is the inside office decor pleasing to you?
- Is the outside decor of the building pleasing to you?
- If the doctor has referred you to a specialist, was the referral acceptable? Please give the name of the specialist referred to: _____ (Again, your confidentiality is assured.)
- Are our fees fair?
- How do you rate the overall quality of care we provide?
- Do you plan to use our offices again when needed. If not, why not? (Again, your confidentiality is assured.)

Game Plan—To find out if your internal marketing is working, modify the above, and duplicate the process. With it, you and your staff can continue to provide quality service, even add new ones and make improvements. From the feedback, identify those areas you need to work on. Sometimes, those areas are you! Make adjustments and then rerun the questionnaire 6 or 12 months later. If you don't check again with the same questions, you'll never know whether you're succeeding or failing.

T.S. found some real eye-openers—longer than acceptable waiting times and a battle-ax on the phone (which seems to be a common problem). Some changes in scheduling and one change at the front desk addressed the problems. His recall percentage increased because of the changes as well as the attitude of caring that the questionnaire projected to all his existing and former patients.

"I never knew you could quantify and control it all. It certainly makes a lot more sense doing it analytically."

☐ NEW HIGHS FOR LOW PATIENT RECALL RATES

N.J., an Illinois gynecologist, called *The Practice Builder* advisory hotline with an urgent request for help. Problem: His recall rate had fallen *below 50%*. The very existence of N.J.'s practice was threatened in the long run if he couldn't retain a much greater percentage of patients.

The Cause—The major culprits behind N.J.'s troubles were his increasingly aggressive competitors. Promotion by start-up obstetricians and gynecologists as well as by established practitioners had become hard hitting. Direct mail and newspaper ads were appearing. The display ad section of his *Yellow Pages* looked like a war zone.

For N.J.'s patients, this meant that between their last appointment and the time for their recall, they were bombarded with temptation—promises of more sensitive care, greater convenience, PMS specialists. Many couldn't resist.

Temptation like this is only tempting if patients view themselves as open to it. Once they've completed a treatment with you or seen you for their periodic examination, they see themselves as "finished." With such a mental ending point, the question of whether to see the same practitioner next time can become an open one, especially with so many competitors blaring so many seemingly good reasons to switch. This is what happened to N.J.

Neutralizing the Competition—But if we remove the "finish," we remove the patient's need to later decide whether to return to you when next in need of an exam or further treatment. By having patients make that decision under good conditions, we prevent patients from being swayed by other competitors.

It's for this reason that a good recall scheduling system can be critical. By having your front desk schedule the recall appointment at the time of the patient's last office visit, the patient then need never decide whether to call for a recall appointment. The decision's already been made. Most are now mentally immune to competitor's persuasive claims.

How To Recall—At the end of the patient's last appointment, set the recall date and time—no matter whether it's 6, 12, or 18 months in advance. Explain that you reserve your most requested times for recall patients. And to assure availability, it's best to pencil in the appointment now. Several weeks before the appointment, you'll send a reminder. Of course, if need be, the time may then be rearranged. But at least this quickly booked-up time will be reserved for that patient.

Agreement to future appointments works well if the appointment is within 12 months. Beyond that, most will decline the offer. But not all, so ask anyway.

If you can't make an appointment for them, have them address a special recall card, one that lists all the reasons why they need to come in for the visit. Send it 4 weeks ahead; their handwriting reminds them that they'd committed for the recall although the date had not been set. If they don't call, your front desk calls to set the appointment.

When you send the recall notice with the scheduled time and date, you're reminding patients of the commitment they've already made. Since they've already made the decision whether to return to you, the only decision is whether the time is still convenient.

Results—How well does it work? "Our recall rate improved 22 percentage points," said N.J. "It seems we worked so hard to get new patients, it hurt when we lost them so easily. But now things have really turned around."

Your first priority should be to work on improving recall percentages *before* any other practice-building activity.

☐ COMPLETE PROGRAM BOOSTS RECALLS

What about the patients who don't schedule their recall appointments at their last visit and don't immediately respond to recall reminders?

If you've ever failed to renew your subscription to *Time* or *Newsweek*, you've been the target of the perfect recall program. Each publication has between 10 and 15 notices prepared and ready to send you until you give in and renew. Both have determined that after a certain point, it's no longer profitable to pursue you. But they've got the numbers to show that until then, if they don't contact you, they're leaving money on the table.

And so it is with the professions. If all you send is one or two postcards in your recall system, you're giving many of your patients away to your competitors. Repetition works here the same as it does elsewhere.

Multistep Program—Consider at least five steps—preferably more—in your recall system. For instance, after sending the initial postcard, have your front desk call to confirm. This reduces no-shows. And it allows your office a chance to answer any objections the patient has. *Always* ask to schedule another appointment when the patient cancels. If you don't ask, you don't get.

Missed appointments should also be called within 15 minutes to ask for a reschedule. If not, you won't be able to train that no-show to keep future appointments.

If the patient still doesn't schedule an appointment, send a letter that you've personally signed. The message: why it's important for the patient to come in now and what the risks are if he or she doesn't. Obviously, the specifics change from specialty to specialty, but you must be specific.

If there's still no response, have the front desk call again. The message is the same: why it's important for the patient to come in and what could happen if he or she doesn't. Then ask for the appointment. Script the conversation so the caller doesn't speak inappropriately. Also have answers to objections ready so the caller is always prepared. If there's still no appointment, recall again a few months later.

Are You Bothering People?—Professionals often raise this question, and it's a valid concern. One must first assume that you're not recalling someone who doesn't need to see you again—that's a breach of your professional ethics. But if they need to be recalled, it's incumbent on you to make sure they have the opportunity *and* that they understand the consequences of not coming in. Are you bothering them? Not if you're recalling those who need to see you.

But recalls can come across as annoying. And they do so only when the communication *feels* self-serving. If you recall someone without solid reasons, *or you fail to convey those reasons*, it will appear that you're doing it only for the business. That's annoying.

So make sure all written and spoken recalls are created with only the patient's concerns in mind. Then it's not annoying or self-serving. It shows concern and caring.

☐ INCREASING YOUR RECALL RATE

Most physicians who need a recall system have one—or at least a semblance of one.

But few have an *optimal* recall system laced with convincing reasons to come back. And one with a fair amount of repetition to make sure all who can return, do so. As seen in the previous article, it should include scheduling the recall at the time of the last appointment, a postcard addressed by the patient in his or her own handwriting, a follow-up call to confirm, plus a series of three to five letters and calls to those who don't respond to your first efforts.

Preconditioning for Recalls—Once that system is in place, it's time to think about ways *not* to use it. The idea, of course, is to have as many patients respond to your first and second efforts, not your third through sixth.

In business, the way most heady people have historically accomplished this in their own industry is by *preconditioning*—by having the person ready for a recall *before* they are recalled. And it can be done in medicine, too. In this way, your patients will have accepted the idea of recalling by the time you've finished their initial service so you needn't convince them later on. This is easier to do in the beginning because people are most receptive when you're working with them but become less receptive when you haven't seen them for 6 to 24 months. Also, face-to-face communication is far more persuasive than a card or phone call. So, in essence, the recall preconditioning should start when you start providing service.

Preconditioning Steps—To get your patients preconditioned for a recall, consider the following:

1. While providing your services, make a number of references to the importance of prevention: "Prevention takes a minute. Correction can never have enough time." "Prevention is always inexpensive, but treatment can be costly."

2. Talk about how the recall is necessary to see how well the current service is working and whether any fine adjustments are required.

3. After you talk about the importance of the recall, make the client *promise* to return so he or she doesn't become one of your tragic cases. (It's amazing how much influence you as an authority figure can wield if you use it constructively.)

4. Get the person to agree on a certain month and time of the month for recall. Explain you're going to help him or her keep that promise. That's part of your job as the gatekeeper of the individual's health care.

5. Send a thank-you note at the end of providing your service that mentions the recall in a specific month. Add a note that you'll definitely check on (name their specific problem) at that time. A word processor is handy for this.

Results—Iowa doctor D.M. used this system in his office and he reports *a 95% response rate*. The figure speaks for itself.

☐ MULTIPLE APPOINTMENT CARDS INCREASE FULFILLMENT

Have you ever suggested that a patient come in for a series of visits, but after the first or second appointment, the patient never returns? The reasons why may vary: inertia; lack of sufficient motivation; or perhaps money. But by applying the same principle discussed above—by having the patient make a firm commitment for the entire course of treatment upfront—you're less likely to see a disappearing act.

Set the Series—Instead of setting only the next appointment at each visit, set the entire series at the first meeting. At this time, commitment is highest. Solidify it by putting *all* of the dates and times on a single appointment card. This visually reinforces and reminds them of their commitment and makes it more difficult to break.

If the patient won't commit to setting appointments, at least set a time frame—for example, from the second through the fourth weeks in May—for the series of visits. Then have the office call later to set up the specific time and date.

To cut down on no-shows, remember to reconfirm each appointment by phone beforehand.

☐ WINNING PRESENTATIONS: THE ONE-MINUTE MESSAGE

A year and a half ago, Dr. H.B., a practitioner in a large New York suburb, decided to try a new idea to develop his practice. His experience told him that if he spent more time listening to his patients, he could uncover a number of needs that he could fill. And the patients were often unaware that they needed the additional service.

The problem was lack of time. To thoroughly engage someone was an impossible luxury in his busy practice. A more streamlined method needed to be developed. In fact, he was searching for an easier way to educate his patients so they could help identify their own needs.

Fostering Awareness—So Dr. H.B. adopted a new, compact, structured way to foster increased patient awareness. Over a 3-month period, he spent one extra minute with each patient discussing one of three health enhancement topics regarding treatments he offered.

He noticed immediate response to each one of his themes. But what he found most impressive were the residual effects. Over a year later, patients were still coming to him for one of his treatment programs, citing his one-minute education as the reason.

The program is now called "thematic promotion." And it proves the power of a professional's verbal recommendation. This program is so successful and flexible that all professionals can adapt it. New developments in a field lend themselves perfectly to thematic promotion, but so do older topics.

Doing the Homework—Choose a topic for which you can provide treatment. Carefully write a script and memorize it. Convey it to each patient in a fluid, natural delivery in under a minute. The topic need not necessarily apply at that moment to that patient. Encourage them to share this information with friends and family as a service.

To avoid duplication of themes, mark each chart that the patient has been informed about "X" theme. After 2 or 3 weeks, discontinue that theme. Rest 2 or 3 weeks and then begin with the next theme. Use your imagination to develop a series of enticing topics that your patients will appreciate and turn to you for treatment.

Results—Dr. P.R. began thematic promotions on a consistent basis over 2 years ago. He reports an increase of 15% in his income directly attributable to his 30 additional seconds with each patient. Many of them call a year later to ask him further questions about one of his themes. He observes, "These thematic promotions are a tremendous way to create awareness of patient needs that I may not even be aware of and that they can now tell me about. And of course, providing additional services to existing patients is easier and less costly than getting new patients."

☐ WIN-WIN PRESENTATIONS

Traditional presentation techniques, designed to overcome objections and to maneuver the patient into saying yes, usually result in an atmosphere of antagonism. And in the long run that's harmful to the practitioner-patient relationship.

But today there's an alternative for the in-tune professional. A technique called "nonmanipulative selling" (NMS) focuses on the patient's problems rather than what you have to offer.[1] Technique: Mentally place yourself in the patient's shoes. Simple in concept, but it takes great concentration in practice.

Physicians often have a choice between recommending more innovative, expensive procedures or proposing more traditional or less expensive intervention. After probing with open-ended questions, one physician understood his patient's conservative nature and recommended the less radical and less costly alternative. "Afterwards, he really thanked me for my understanding. He said he mistrusted doctors because two others had insisted he needed a more costly treatment, and he thought they were greedy. By listening, I was able to give what he needed *and* wanted. Now, he's not only a loyal patient, but he's one of my biggest supporters with eight referrals in 18 months."

☐ USING QUESTIONS TO GAIN COMMITMENTS

Most physicians make their recommendations and then just hope for the best. There's a better way, according to The Dartnell Corporation,[2] one of the world's largest firms in the business of teaching presentation skills. Practitioners should gain minicommitments—the patient agreeing with your points—all along the way. "Gain three or more commitments from the patient, and they have to say yes."

Why Questions?—First, if you ask a question and obtain a positive answer, you've gotten a minicommitment. That puts the patient on record. The more agreements along the way, the more the likelihood of an agreement at the close.

Secondly, questions can be stronger than statements. Strong statements don't ask patients to decide. But statements with "don't you agree?" or "isn't it?" at the end do. They create stronger results because the patient's decision making on that point has been voiced.

Examples: "Don't you think it would be better to take care of it now and not have to think about it anymore?" "From my analysis, I feel this is the best alternative of the three. Don't you agree?" "This looks like the best value, doesn't it?"

You'll notice that many of these examples are simply positive statements with an "isn't it?" or "aren't they?" added at the end to gain the commitment.

To Gain More Commitments—Use words that require a positive response wherever possible, such as "do you understand how this . . . ?" or "wouldn't you like . . . ?" or "don't you feel . . . ?" or "do you appreciate that . . . ?"

Yet beware of using the word "convince." People automatically put up their guard when trying to be convinced or sold. Better strategy: Let them be the judge. There's no resistance when you encourage people to exercise power and control.

Key Point—Most times you need three or more minicommitments before the close when you ask for the patient's overall decision about your recommendation.

☐ SEVERAL OTHER PRESENTATION TACTICS

When making presentations, there are some aspects of human nature that you should be aware of so your own behavior or thinking

☐ **The 3-3-3 Formula in Presentation Tactics**

When a patient asks why he or she should say yes to your recommendation, chances are you could ramble off one or two good reasons. But Charles Lapp,[3] professor of business at Drake University, says that's not enough. Lapp advises practitioners to be prepared with reasons why patients should use your services—not those of a colleague—and why they should use your services *now*.

The 3-3-3 Formula—Prepare three reasons to buy, three reasons to buy from you, and three reasons to buy from you now. By preparing these ahead of time, you avoid the pitfalls of shooting from the hip and looking as if you're having a hard time coming up with good reasons.

___

or your patient's natural behavior doesn't unwittingly stand in the way of the best course of action.

1. *Offer your best recommendation first.* When presenting multiple courses of action to patients, keep in mind that 90% of the patients will accept the alternative you give first, no matter whether you believe another option is better. So offer your best recommendation first.
2. *Use the right tone.* Most people respond to a low-key, gentle approach. Avoid being glib. In making presentations, speak slower than normal, stick with plain language, not technical terms, and don't be too friendly or open at first.
3. *Overcome your fear of closings.* Most physicians dislike asking a patient to spend a sizable amount of money. This fear of asking for a commitment at the close of a presentation stems from a sense that the person is being asked for a favor.
4. *Change your perspective.* Recognize that the person needs you. Take it for granted. Remember the benefits you're offering. Rather than ask if they want to go through with your recommendation, simply ask if now or next week would be best to start.

☐ **OBJECTION CLINIC**

While all of the above techniques increase the likelihood that your recommendation will be accepted, you will still encounter objections. Let's look at the most common objections and how they can be countered.

■ Objection: "It Costs Too Much"

Everybody's talking price. More and more practitioners face price objections daily, even from established patients. "It costs too much." "The price is too high."

But there are sound tactics to handle these objections easily and profitably. Properly schooled, the average practitioner can overcome two to three times as many price objections as before. Here's how.

Analyze before answering. Find out what the patient really means. "Too high in what respect?" Such questions help you decide how to answer this objection. Does the patient know you're offering good value for your price? Does he or she know what the procedure you're recommending can do for them? Find out.

Apples to Oranges—Differentiate your services from lower-priced ones. The same procedure offered by another doctor is not the same as the one performed by you. You have more training, more experience, more advanced techniques, your unsurpassed staff, and so forth. This same differentiation also defeats competition from nonmedical alternatives.

Say, "I know you can probably buy for less. You can always buy lower. But I wonder if we are talking about exactly the same thing. Let's take a minute to find out, shall we?" Then compare and distinguish your services from the competition.

Form-Fitting Tactics—Once you know the basis for the objection and have the patient's cooperation, choose the best fitting tactics:

1. Emphasize value: What your service means to the patient. "Our service does this for you "*so that* you'll have/you'll feel/ you'll be . . . " *So that* are the key words. That phrase introduces the benefits that the patient should be weighing.
2. Emphasize quality: Compare your offering to the lower-priced offering.
3. Emphasize dependability: Cite your success rate, longevity of the benefits, and the like.
4. Emphasize exclusive advantages: What you offer that others don't.
5. Emphasize follow-up services: This will always differentiate you since even though many do it, few talk about it.

More Methods—One physician asks the patient, "How many years do you figure you'll benefit from this service?" When given an answer, the doctor breaks down the price to a daily cost and uses this to show how little the extra value received actually costs.

Use visuals. Telling something isn't enough to convince. Dramatize through demonstration. Show results of tests, studies, or experience as revealed through case histories and testimonials. Emphasize the longevity of the benefits the patient will receive and the satisfaction others already have.

Use words that motivate. Dry language means objections remain. Instead, pepper your presentation with words that describe legitimate qualities yet also distinguish it: new, extra, larger, longer, quicker, proven. They make any price seem more reasonable.

Remember: First, understand the objection from the patient's point of view. Second, stress the value vs. the price of the service. Emphasize your higher quality of care, dependability, exclusive advantages, and better service. If need be, break down the price to a daily, monthly, or yearly figure.

These methods add up to better value and can be appraised in terms of "worth more" to convince and overcome the price objection.

■ Objection: "I'll Think It Over"

Every physician makes recommendations at times only to have the patient balk by saying, "I'll think it over." This isn't an objection; it's a put off. And the patient is avoiding telling you the real objection.

Instead, pin the patient down so you can tackle the real objection that lies behind the evasion. Ask, "Is there something about the recommendation that doesn't exactly suit you?" or "Do you mind telling me why you want to wait?"

If you don't know the real objection, you can't resolve it.

■ Objection: "I Can't Afford It"

It isn't unusual for patients to react to your recommendations with the plea that they can't afford the course of action you've proposed. Pleading poverty doesn't always mean the patient is poor—only that your presentation might be.

What the patient is really saying is "the benefits of your services don't seem worth the cost to me, given what I could be spending that money on." If the patient really wanted what you recommended, other competing discretionary purchases would be seen as a poor second place.

So the first step in answering this objection is to restate the benefits of the prescribed course. What will it do for the patient? What will the patient risk by not going ahead with it? Why should the procedure be done now? In a word—benefits. Lots and lots of benefits. The more impressive the benefits and the more importance given to them, the more acceptance.

☐ **Perle Mesta's Secret to Patient Retention**

Someone once asked Perle Mesta, the greatest Washington hostess since Dolly Madison, for the secret of her success in getting so many rich and famous people to attend her parties. "It's all in the greetings and good-byes," she answered. As each person arrived, she would meet him or her with "at last you're here!" And as each guest left, she expressed her regrets with "I'm sorry you have to leave so soon!"

The more important you make someone feel, the more loyalty you inspire.

But what happens if the objection still stands even though your presentation has been convincing? In this case, money is a true objection. So make the unaffordable affordable by offering terms—so much down, so much per week or month.

And if the objection still stands, consider taking less money, but not lowering the price. To do so, offer one of the limited number of grants the practice makes to help patients get the services they need. The patient pays a reduced fee. The grant from the practice makes up the remainder. The price is maintained so the value of the service in the patient's eyes is also maintained. And the grant approach avoids the problem of price cutting while giving you the flexibility, at times, to price compete.

☐ **PRESENT PROFITS FROM PAST PATIENTS**

Texas psychiatrist L.M. had 400 former patients whom she hadn't seen in 2 years or more. When her schedule slowed, she wrote them a two-page letter. In it, she emphasized that if they were feeling unhappy, unsure, had difficulty sleeping, eating, or communicating, or were overstressed from work or home, perhaps now was the time to get back on track. After all, they had done it once. Perhaps all they needed now was a minor adjustment.

Results: Sixteen patients returned, plus four new referrals from past patients. Total: a 5% response to the mailing.

It's a shrewd strategy because it's easier to convince your previous patients to purchase services from you again than to attract new ones with whom you've had no established relationship.

REFERENCES

1. Alessandra AJ: *Nonmanipulative Selling*. Reston, VA, Reston Publishing Co, 1984.
2. *Salesmanship*, The Dartnell Corporation, 4660 Ravenswood Ave, Chicago, IL 60640, 1986, p 5.
3. Frank W, Lapp C: *How to Outsell the Born Salesman*, New York, Collier Books, 1972, p 87.

■ CHAPTER 7
Gaining Referrals From Patients And Staff
More Easily Still

☐ CAN I REALLY ASK FOR REFERRALS?

Some very revealing information was uncovered from a survey commissioned by the nation's major charities to find out why people give. When people were asked why they give to charity, the reason most often given was *not* because it was a worthy cause, *not* because of tax reasons, and *not* because of guilt. The most common answer was that they gave because they were *asked to give*.

For charities, this means they don't have to have fancy strategies. They just have to organize lots of people to do the asking.

For professionals, this behavioral trait also has great implications. It means that all you have to do to increase referrals from existing patients is to ask. Ask everyone. And it doesn't cost anything.

Untapped Asset—If you questioned professionals about referrals, most of them would tell you that their greatest source of referrals are their own patients. And yet they assume all of their patients know their practice is open. However, according to a recent *Practice Builder* survey, 31% of the patients queried did not believe their practitioner was accepting new patients. And a full 43% said they didn't know one way or the other.

What to do?

Two Remedies—Signs in the waiting room can do the job. "We appreciate and especially welcome new patients." You can also incorporate a message into your newsletter and other promotional vehicles. It might read as follows:

> Yes, We are Accepting New Patients
> Our patients often ask if we are accepting additional patients. We're happy to say yes. We very much appreciate your referrals. When you send us a patient, you can be certain they'll be treated with our best efforts to justify the faith you've placed in us. I assure you that you'll feel proud you did.
>
> (Your signature)

But the simplest method of getting new referrals, of course, is to follow the lead of the charities—ask. Most physicians, however, find this difficult to do, understandably so, until they try it once or twice. Try it. "It's been a pleasure helping you. And if you have someone just as nice as you, please send them to us. I'd appreciate it."

Results—Dr. S.S. felt uncomfortable at first in asking his patients for referrals. As time went on, however, his requests became smoother and more relaxed. And a referral sign went up in the waiting room. After 6 months, patient referrals had doubled. Each referrer was sent a letter of appreciation, while heavy referrers were awarded gifts such as flowers, wine, or books.

"I found out my patients are the greatest assets of my practice, and I've been overlooking them all these years. No more—not with results like these."

☐ REWARDING REFERRALS: WHO DOES WHAT?

As a rule of thumb, 80% of referrals come from 20% of the patients. Figures may vary, but the pattern of the many from the few is almost universal. Therefore, it follows that professionals should encourage those already referring to refer even more—or at least to keep the referrals coming at the same pace. Consequently, a practitioner should have an organized process to identify, thank, and generally treat heavy referrers with special care.

To find out whether this is the case, *The Practice Builder* conducted a telephone survey with 116 professionals. The findings were as follows:

- 90.5% did not maintain or could not compile a list of those who refer heavily
- 62% did not in any way thank referrers

- Of the 38% who did thank their referrers, only about one in ten of the sample did anything special for multiple referrers.

Not very impressive.

Key Elements—A good program of rewarding referrers capitalizes on the fact that often your existing patients have friends, family, and neighbors who are your primary targets. The program also capitalizes on the basic precepts of Psych 101—you can shape referring behavior by reinforcing it. Use recognition, praise, personal attention, gifts, or monetary incentives. Write cards, call personally, send a plant or bottle of wine, provide a dinner at a local restaurant, or offer a free office visit.

The survey confirms that so few professionals do anything at all, any recognition will go a long way. Better yet, a good program will demonstrate that internal promotion can be very high powered.

☐ REFERRALS FROM UNEXPECTED PLACES

Orthopedic surgeon D.S. received seven referrals from a single patient in just 60 days. After every referral, he sent a thank you note, even a plant, then wine, and finally a basket filled with fruit, cheese, and wine. On the seventh referral, he figured he should call and thank the patient personally. Lucky for him he did.

D.S. discovered the patient worked as a manicurist in a hair salon. And the people she referred were all her clients whom she had given pedicures. Makes sense, doesn't it?

Being quick to realize the potential, D.S. mailed an invitation to all the manicurists in the area in care of each of the town's hair salons requesting their attendance at a special *free* seminar on how to recognize and deal with clients who have foot problems. The motivation: an appeal to the manicurists' desire to become *more professional* in their calling and overcome their sense of inferiority. Also to give them a "leg up" on their competition.

At the seminar, D.S. gave enough information in an hour and a half for the eight attendees to know *when to refer* to an orthopedic surgeon. He also conducted examinations on everyone there to further display his abilities. He also gave out his practice brochures and plenty of business cards.

At the end of the seminar, he suggested that when appropriate, the manicurists always refer their clients to a qualified orthopedic surgeon. And if they wanted their clients to see D.S., he'd be sure to give them special attention if the client mentioned the manicurist's name when calling for the appointment.

Three Big Questions for Move-Ins—When a family moves to a new area, the wife and mother usually tracks down the people to fill three roles: the family physician, the dentist, and her hairdresser. Typically, she sees the hairdresser more often than the doctor or dentist, so she'll find the beautician first. And because it takes time for a family who's moved to meet neighbors and other possible referrers, it's not surprising that hairdressers can be a *big* source of referrals.

How can you tap into this market? Simple. Contact hairdressers by mail and invite them to a seminar in your office. Follow up your invitation with a phone call. Many more will now attend. Always appeal to their sense of wanting to be seen as a "professional." Teach them when to refer. Exhibit your skills on them since this is always impressive. And give them plenty of promotional material to take to their shops.

Results—An ophthalmologist began a program to promote his permanent eyeliner, radial keratotomy, and collagen therapy procedures through salons. He held seminars at hair salon trade shows in his area, promoting them with big ads in the preshow publicity mailings and in the show directory. His results: over 200 attendees in 4 seminars. "There's quite a bit of discussion about cosmetics in hair salons. So it seemed a natural extension for the stylists to be versed in cosmetic eye surgery also. The seminars gave us instant awareness."

☐ 15% GROWTH—FROM YOUR RECEPTIONIST

In almost every office, the receptionist is among the least skilled and the poorest paid of the entire staff. But in today's leaner times, the marketing-oriented professional is more likely to question this traditional practice by asking, "Why is the staff person who creates that first and longest-lasting impression also the worker who's the least skilled, least trained, and lowest paid?" It no longer makes sense.

Today's Answer—Hire for personality and voice, not experience. Warmth and concern are the key personal attributes your receptionist must exude. When applicants for the receptionist position first call, interview them by phone. If you cannot feel the concern, the smile, the caring, don't bother interviewing them in person.

A pleasant, interested voice combined with a positive attitude is rare. Expect that 85% of your applicants will not meet these standards and shouldn't be considered. Of the remaining 15%, half will have a strong financial motivation. Those with an intense desire to earn are more conscientious and more apt to concentrate on the task at hand.

The Eight Steps to Success—Teach your receptionist the following telephone techniques for success:

1. Talk with callers, not at them. Concentrate on each caller's main concern—himself.
2. Isolate each call; forget the last call. Treat each as if it were the only call received all day.
3. Pause after each sentence. This adds importance to what you say.
4. Vary the tone and pitch of your voice naturally. Tonight, listen to the TV announcer and observe the result of years of training and practice.
5. Lower the volume of your voice at the end of most sentences without going downhill with the tone of your voice.
6. Enunciate clearly. This will not only improve voice quality but also your credibility.
7. Smile! It will be transmitted in your voice and do all the work for you.
8. There is no rush, not when it comes to patients.

Train, Then Manage—Explain to your receptionist the importance of the position to you and to the entire team. Tell your receptionist exactly what you expect in performance, and write these goals down on one page. Inform your VIR (very important receptionist) that you'll be monitoring the office phone calls to offer pointers to improve his or her performance. Clear goals and immediate praising and reprimanding are the keys to successful management.

Monitoring is of the utmost importance. A successful physician must weed out as soon as possible those not willing to do what is expected of them. Each day that an unsuitable person remains in the receptionist position, the greater the number of poor impressions created, and the weaker the entire structure of your staff becomes.

Proven Results—For years, Dr. H.G. had employed a technically competent but rather cold—and sometimes testy—receptionist. She kept the office running smoothly but nothing else. Finally, he accidentally overheard a conversation that his receptionist handled mildly inappropriately. She did not do enough damage to upset anyone, but she certainly did nothing to surpass the patient's expectations.

Realizing that he wouldn't want to be treated that way himself,

☐ **Caution: Your Staff Can Torpedo Marketing Plans**

Before you implement a new marketing program, make sure your staff doesn't sabotage it. Why would they? All of us resist changes. Changes cause stress that affects productivity and the staff's conduct. Without your staff's support, your new program is doomed even before it starts.

Tackle that resistance by giving your staff advance notice of the changes. After all, much of their resistance arises from deep fears that their routines and security will be threatened. Solicit their suggestions. Calm their fears.

Dr. H.G. mustered up his courage and replaced the receptionist. He hired the most caring and mature individual he could find, trained her intensely, set out goals, and gave immediate praise when due, as well as reprimands.

With her personality and his instruction, she converted more shoppers to patients in 1 week than the former receptionist did in a month. The practice grew more than 15% with no other changes. Her caring attitude told prospective patients to expect the same kind of care from her employer.

☐ **NEW INCENTIVES FOR MARKETING BY YOUR STAFF**

As suggested in Chapters 5 and 6, to pinpoint problems you can survey former patients to find out why they left your care, but that's not enough. By itself, it's like driving the practice by looking through the rearview mirror. Instead of just detecting mistakes and then fixing them, prevent them by having your staff treat every patient the way you would.

Incentives—Consider the newest type of staff incentive program. It's an old idea in business, but few professionals have tried it, even though it works well for them. For example, Dr. L.J. in Wisconsin reports an average monthly growth of 13% since he started a staff incentive plan. "Everyone tries really hard now. They're all concerned so they act concerned. And we're functioning together like a committed team. That wasn't so before."

In the past, a professional might set an arbitrary monthly goal— perhaps 15% over last year. If the goal was met, the staff would divide up some percentage of the growth, say 3%. But if the performance fell short of that mark and reached only 12%, then no bonus was paid.

Another Approach—It's better to use a graduated incentive scale. Construct it so that the higher the productivity, the higher *the percentage* of growth the staff receives. The more the practice makes, the more they make. Key: Inform them of the practice receipts during the month. Keep the updated targets and totals for the month near the coffee pot.

To have your staff recruit patients, set up another program. Print business cards for staff members, and encourage them to pass out those cards to friends, neighbors, family, and business acquaintances. For each patient referred by a staff member, pay the incentive. Give an additional incentive if the referred patient spends over $X. Reinforce the big cases.

Money Isn't Everything—These days, money isn't always the best incentive. If the staff receives it this week, it's gone the next. But if you give a TV, they talk about it for years. The recognition lasts, and the staff member thinks fondly of you long afterwards.

Choose merchandise incentives for lower rewards and travel for larger ones. Weekend trips are good intermediates. From $25 to $1,000, the possibilities are endless—books, cookware, cameras, calculators, clocks, sporting goods, giftware, silverware, VCRs, compact disk players. Extra vacation time also motivates nicely.

Write for what's called a plateau catalog. It's divided into price sections to let employees choose any item from a specific plateau. Different plateaus reflect different costs. How do you find a plateau catalog? Look in the *Yellow Pages* of a large metropolitan area for companies that specialize in incentive programs.

Today, incentive programs are even used to reduce absenteeism. Try them for anything that's measurable. Why? Because incentives work and *they pay for themselves.*

■ CHAPTER 8
Practice Brochures And Newsletters: Step-By-Step Do's And Dont's Plus A Big Warning

☐ PRACTICE BROCHURES: THE BEST GAME PLAN

There was never any question whether Maryland dermatologist R.C. should have a practice brochure. Everyone told him that to generate more business, he needed one. All the literature said so too.

So he had 5,000 printed with no expense spared; he had it done on heavy paper with two folds, printed in three colors, and embossed—a quality look. The brochure included a dry discussion of dermatologic treatment in general, a biographical sketch, information about how to have one's questions answered and make payment arrangements, a list of office policies, and the doctor's name, address, and phone number.

Now what? Conventional wisdom said to give it to all prospective patients and send it to all existing ones. So R.C. did. But the business he expected from the brochure just didn't materialize.

Someone then suggested that he mail the brochure to upper middle-income families with zip codes near his office. Game plan: 10,000 brochures, each mailed without any other enclosures. Result: total disappointment.

Producing a practice brochure because someone or everyone said so made R.C. fall flat on his face. What seemed a good idea wasn't, because he didn't start out by answering a couple of basic questions: who's the piece intended for, and what specifically should it accomplish? Without asking those questions and having good answers, R.C.'s brochure was doomed before it was written.

The Right Game Plan—If R.C. were to produce a brochure for new patients, then the brochure needn't convince them to come in. But it must reinforce the idea that they chose the right practitioner to overcome the buyer's remorse or postpurchase dissonance—the second guessing that takes place after a prospective patient has committed to coming initially but hasn't necessarily committed to coming for good. The brochure can help calm their fears by making all those complimentary points that would sound like bragging if the practitioner were to say them.

The brochure should also be a recital of office policies—a simple fact sheet of hours, payment policies, fees, and so on. The "riot act" information can also be included in this sheet: What happens if the patient misses an appointment, when payment is due and all the negative points you don't particularly want to discuss before the patient walks through the door or for that matter, face-to-face. Money spent on an exotic layout and expensive printing doesn't pay here.

But if R.C. wants the brochure to interest and convince prospective patients, then it must be sales oriented—why choose R.C. over other dermatologists? What do the benefits mean to a patient? It must have a strong biographical sketch with examples of successes and a menu of services the doctor provides with no mention of office policies. Everything in the brochure sells, or it doesn't go in.

That includes the cover. When selling, the cover has a headline with a benefit stated or implied. The practice name may be on the cover or may be inside with the address, phone number, and logo. But the practice name is not a headline.

Also include a tear-out business reply card to request more information. The more ways you give to respond, the more response you get.

Production of this type of brochure is where your resources should be spent. Put your money in the art direction for a strong visual impact, its copywriting, photography, printing, and paper. Creation of the right image is your primary concern.

How to Use It—The brochure serves as a handout when making presentations to prospective patients. If the patient doesn't make a commitment during the first appointment, the selling brochure is taken home to reinforce the points made during the consultation. And even when the prospective patient has made a commitment, the brochure is given out to calm the new patient's postpurchase dissonance.

The sales brochure also serves as a handout at your speeches and seminars. It provides more information about you that could sound like bragging if you were to say it yourself. And it makes an additional impression to reinforce your personal one.

More Uses—As described in Chapter 7, if you have an incentive program for your staff to help promote the practice, the brochure professionally delivers a message in a way the staff can't match. Along with your business card, the sales brochure is the perfect handout.

Want to save money? Create a selling brochure to act as your main promotional piece. Then print a separate insert and other "riot act" information. Voilà. Your selling piece now becomes your patient information brochure, nicely calming buyer's remorse and at the same time enabling you to avoid the need for two brochure layouts and printing runs.

At times the selling brochure can be used as a direct mail piece. But never all by itself. Always use a cover letter, written in a more personal style than the brochure, in which you can highlight specific benefits over and over again.

However, the brochure may not be the best marketing piece to use in direct mail. Here again, first define the goal and the mailing strategy. Then design the best direct-mail package for top results. Consider yourself fortunate if the brochure does happen to fill the need. Most practice brochures don't.

The Right Approach—Decide your purpose, define you goal, design your strategy. Then create the brochure you need.

☐ Practice Brochure Analysis: Benefits Galore

The cover of the practice brochure shown in Figure 8–1 is obviously intended to convince prospective patients that they've found the right practice in this psychiatrist and psychologist team. There's no beating around the bush about the benefit conveyed in the cover's headline, "Have the life you want."

As seen in Figure 8–2, the three inside panels set out to forcefully make two points. First, here are two professionals who care. The brochure doesn't try to persuade readers that psychiatry or psychology deserve their consideration. Only that Drs. Ross and Covert do. Second, much of the copy reinforces and expands on the benefit on the cover. Over and over, the copy conveys that help is at hand: "Set satisfying goals . . . and reach them." "Tomorrow can be better—with the right help." "You *can* have the life you want."

On the back panels, shown in Figure 8–3, is a call to action with the practice's phone number. The brochure concludes with a panel devoted to biographic sketches of the two practitioners.

Everything in the brochure has been placed there for a purpose—to promote the practice and address the concerns of a prospective patient. Well done.

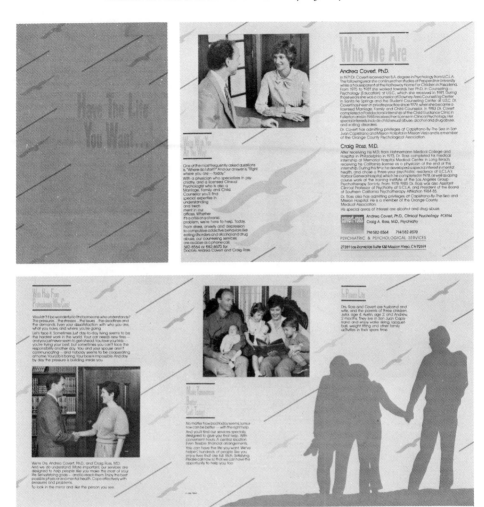

FIGS 8–1 (top left), 8–2 (bottom), and 8–3 (top right).

☐ HOW TO PRODUCE A HANDOUT QUICKLY, EASILY, AND CHEAPLY

Brochures to educate, convince, announce, or recruit? Flyers for seminars or announcements? Or a thousand other purposes? How can you produce them "quick and dirty" and still have them look professional, especially when the purpose is short term or not so important as to warrant more expensive production?

Simple. Just follow this recipe. In terms of brochures and flyers, it's easy. Well, it may not be *easy* if you haven't done one before, but it is much easier today than in the past. These steps should make it easier still:

1. *Don't start writing; decide your format first.* Writing to a predetermined format will force you to write the right amount of copy. So fit the writing to the format, not the other way around. For example, you might decide on a $8^1/_2 \times 11$-in. brochure printed on both sides, folded in thirds to fit a no. 10 business envelope. Or perhaps one 11 $\times$ 17-in. sheet folded in half to make a four-page $8^1/_2 \times 11$-in. handout. Once you decide on the flyer size, draw in pencil what will go where: headline, pictures, drawings, masthead, and so on. Now you know how much to write.

2. *Outline.* Make a short outline and put down your points in order. Does the progression make sense? Big mistakes in thinking are often uncovered right here.

3. *Write.* Short words, short sentences, short paragraphs. No $25 words. Just plain English.

4. *Edit.* Because *no one* writes it right the first time through.

5. *The next day, edit again.* Because *no one* writes it right the second time either.

6. *Send it to the computerized layout house.* With desktop publishing spreading everywhere, shops now exist where you can take your golden prose and the next day have a brochure ready for the printer. These new businesses have Apple, Hewlett Packard, or IBM desktop publishing systems and a laser printer to produce your material cheaply—$50 to $100 to lay out a brochure *including typesetting*. Call your local computer shop, and ask who's got desktop printing equipment in your area.

7. *Send it to the quick printer.* In addition to saving on typesetting, let's save on printing too. Sixty-pound offset paper—white or colored—or something with a light texture like laid (watermarked with fine lines running across the grain) will do well. For these jobs, there's no need to use more than two colors; one color will often do. But don't use photocopying—that's tacky.

"Welcome to our office" informational brochures lend themselves well to this production scheme. Open house invitations, special in-house "take one" promotions, coupons, and newsletters are also prime candidates.

So next time you have a brochure or flyer to produce, spare the staff and yourself the production agony. Cook it up quickly and send it out. And the cost will be less than a trip to your gastroenterologist for the ulcer.

☐ Rx FOR BORING NEWSLETTERS

Six months ago, Pennsylvania pediatrician R.A. sent out his first patient newsletter. He'd worked almost 6 weeks researching the *right* material and constructing his articles. Then he supervised layout, pasteup, printing, and mailing. Results: Nothing. Not even one parent mentioned the newsletter.

The greatest problem for practice newsletters like R.A.'s is that they bore the reader. No, to be more accurate, most never get that far because if they look boring, they're not even read.

Since their authors can't view their work objectively, they think they've created a bible of information. So the physician cranks out more boring prose in the next issue, which is even less likely to be read because the patient now knows what to expect.

Why Most Newsletters Are Boring—They're written like term papers. This is understandable since practitioners have only written in college or during their professional training. In those halcyon days, dry writing was honored, the passive voice revered. And if you described a person, you left your emotions out of it. Just the facts, please.

But now in writing for different readers, the style has to change. To get your newsletter read and passed around, do what the pros do. Write about people. Proof? Look for the most dog–eared magazine in your waiting room. Chances are it's *People*. People love to read about people.

When writing about a new breakthrough, lead with a human interest story or case history. End with what it can mean to the reader. It's more interesting to read about people than ideas. Write about real-life stories, and from these make your point.

Results—Despite an initial failure, Dr. R.A. decided to publish a second issue. Before printing, he rewrote all of his articles, leading each with a story, an example, or an illustration. From those he made his points.

In the first week after its mailing, about 10% of his patients' parents mentioned what a wonderful newsletter he'd written. He received such comments as: "It's really interesting," "I have the same problem as the mother you described in that first story." Visability was achieved. The newsletter is now a valuable practice builder.

☐ TWELVE WAYS TO GET YOUR NEWSLETTER READ

With all the mail people receive, it's difficult to get your newsletter read. And if it's not read, all your hard work goes into the round file.

Well, to make your newsletter readable and increase your response, here are guaranteed tips from Barbara Mehlman,[1] former editor of *Madison Avenue* and copywriter at one of the world's largest ad agencies, Ogilvy & Mather Inc.

■ Improving The Writing

- *Edit out jargon*: Jargon makes writing difficult to understand and boring.
- *Be conversational*: Write as if you were talking to a colleague or friend.
- *Read your writing aloud*: Close your office door, and read your copy aloud to see how it really sounds. If the tone isn't right, you'll hear it. If the sentences don't flow, you'll know it immediately. If you used mixed metaphors, you'll choke on them. If you trip over a tongue twisting combination of words, so will your readers.
- *Let the writing rest*: Let the finished piece sit for a few days so you can judge it more objectively. When you later take a fresh look at it, you'll clearly see flaws you overlooked before, and solutions will likely come to mind.

■ Illustrate Graphically

- *Use charts and pictures with captions*: You don't have room for a thousand words, but you can put in photos.
- *Use short words, short sentences, short paragraphs:* Short means understandable, easy to read. Long means lost.
- *Use subheads*: In longer articles, they break up the tedium. Subheads pick up the pace and add punch.

■ Write Graphically

- *Add zip to headlines*: "How To . . . " "New," "Free" "New Breakthrough Can Change Your . . . " Learn from *Family Circle* and *Glamour*. Any publication that can write headlines for 44 different articles about chocolate cake—all interesting—deserves study.
- *Be specific*: Make your information *usable*, and people will call you for your newsletter.

- *Resist reporting staff events*: Don't write about a staff member's new baby or your vacation. Unless you can show how this information will benefit your readers, don't bore them with it. Actually, you won't have a chance to bore them—they won't read it.

■ Production Tips That Dramatize

- *Type, don't typeset, the newsletter*: Typewriting has a sense of news and urgency. Ragged right edges of columns also add to the feeling.
- *Add importance and variety* with

Boxed articles

Lots of quotes
Bold type
CAPITAL LETTERS
• Bullets
↑ Arrows
Checkmarks √
Underlining
—Dashes
And lists such as these.

■ Other Uses

If these simple ideas will improve your writing and make your newsletter readable, they'll also improve the readability and interest of just about anything else you write to promote your practice.

☐ CLEARING UP FOGGY NEWSLETTERS

Minnesota physician B.P. had had a similar poor response to his practice newsletter. When he asked patients if they had liked it, most embarrassingly answered that they hadn't yet had a chance to read it. This was 2 months after it had been sent. Wondering why, he sent the newsletter to *The Practice Builder* for analysis.

The Findings—The content was interesting enough. But dry, multisyllabic writing made the piece almost unreadable. Even his med school profs might have been left in the fog. Certainly, no one would read it for pleasure.

B.P. Could try to simplify his writing, but how would he know if he was on target? In fact, there's a way to gauge the readability of any writing—including your practice newsletter. Called the "fog index,"[2] it was developed in the 1940s by Robert Gunning to help textbook writers determine how much education it took to understand their writing. And today's practitioners can analyze the complexity of their own writing.

The Fog Index—First, select a passage of 100 to 125 words. Count the number of total words and the number of sentences in the passage. Divide the number of sentences into the number of words to find the average number of words per sentence. That's the sentence length.

Second, count the number of words with three or more syllables. Don't include (1) capitalized words, (2) verb forms made into three syllables with the addition of an "es" or an "ed" such as "divided," or (3) combinations of short and easy words made into a longer word, like "manpower" or "inasmuch."

Once you've got that number of long words, divide it by the total words, and multiply the answer by 100. Add this number to the figure you calculated earlier for sentence length. Finally multiply that sum by 0.4.

That number is the fog index of the writing and indicates the number of years of education a reader must have to decipher your writing. Ignore any decimals in the answer. And anything over 17, just call 17+ since this means a reader needs more than a college education to understand it.

Fogless Writing—Here are the findings by the Gunning-Mueller Clear Writing Institute, which analyzed the writing found in publications today.

PUBLICATION	FOG INDEX (YR OF EDUCATION NEEDED TO READ EASILY)
People	6
Ladies Home Journal	8
Reader's Digest	9–10
Newsweek	11
Time	11
Wall Street Journal	11
Harper's	12
Harvard Business Journal	17+
Dr. B.P.'s Newsletter	17+
This Book	10

No writing can be commercially successful if it averages over 20 words per sentence. *Time, Newsweek,* and *The Wall Street Journal* all average 16 words per sentence.

☐ Nine Ways to Use Your Practice Newsletter

Newsletters have been traditionally used to solidify patient loyalty. Here are some newer, more productive ways to use it:

1. Mail your practice newsletter 1 month prior to sending out your customary recall notices. Repetition of your message can increase response.

2. Or enclose the newsletter with your recall reminders.

3. Or print your recall reminder on the newsletter.

4. If available, enclose appropriate manufacturers' flyers with the newsletter.

5. Use your newsletter as a statement stuffer.

6. Mail your newsletter at least three or four times a year to all present and *past* patients.

7. Mail to the surrounding community to generate new patient flow—but check your state laws for any restrictions.

8. Mail to specific audiences you've identified as prime targets in the community. For example, senior citizen groups, fraternal or religious organizations, sports clubs, and the like.

9. Swap patient or client lists with allied but noncompeting professionals, and mail your newsletter to patients on those lists. Such proven buyers of allied services are preferred prospects.

Also use active words in a conversational tone. Create pictures with them. And always write to express, not to impress.

☐ INCREASING NEWSLETTER READERSHIP

Dr. M.L. saw little response after mailing each of three successive issues of her practice newsletter. Her fear was that the newsletter was being "roundfiled" even though it was well written. What to do?

Incentive Reading—To spur readership, she added a special incentive. Boxed in big letters on page one were the instructions for her newsletter contest. Those readers who found their names in the newsletter could claim a free office visit as the prize. Three names were contained in each issue—good odds that generated a good response.

After her next issue, all three patients called to claim their prize. More than ten other patients said they wished they'd won.

The result was a newsworthy newsletter, both read and responded to.

☐ THE BIG WARNING: WHY NEWSLETTERS OFTEN DON'T WORK; WHAT TO DO INSTEAD

Do you still find your patient newsletter doesn't make your phone ring enough after all the agony of writing it, arguing with the printer, and forcing the staff to lick 3,000 stamps? If it's any consolation, that's true for most newsletter-writing physicians today.

Sometimes no matter how good the copy, it doesn't do the trick, even after sharpening the articles, focusing more on people to make it lively, and sprinkling it with snappy graphics.

The Newsletter Fallacy—Time honored "wisdom" argues that your newsletter ensures that your patients will remember you when they need you; that when they reenter the market for your services, they'll be spurred to call you rather than another physician.

But if that's the case, shouldn't at least some of your existing base need your services when the newsletter arrives? Therefore, it should motivate *additional* patients to call *now*.

However, most newsletters don't. The phones stay fairly quiet. The number of existing patients you see remains steady. Not even a blip on the graph.

If a newsletter can't make the phone ring immediately, how can it make the phone ring several months later? That's the newsletter fallacy.

Why Newsletters Don't Work—Consider this: If when you arrived home this evening you found a telegram, a letter sent first-class, and a newsletter, which would you open first? Chances are you'd open and read them in that order. In fact, each could contain the same information worded in the same way. But the format—the packaging—dictates the priority. The different packages convey different degrees of importance, so it influences our behavior.

Why don't newsletters work? Because there are so many other seemingly more important items to read in the mail that they *can't compete well.* More often than not, they just don't get read, or they are read only if time permits.

New Packaging—Savvy practitioners are now beginning to use this new understanding. They're repackaging their newsletter information into a format that says, "this is important!" So they're turning unread material into internal promotions that grab more attention—immediately.

One packaging alternative is a multipage letter. Mailed on office stationery with either a precancelled bulk stamp or a postage meter cancellation, the mailing looks first class, but the third-class postage costs 37.5% less.

Personalizing the Letter—If possible, print the patient's name and address directly on the envelope, not on a label. A label signals an impersonal communication because they're so often used in commercial direct mail and therefore are of lesser importance. With the stamp and the lack of label, the impression is of an important, official letter from one's physician.

The letter might begin:

> Dear Patient,
>   Here's a problem. There are always new breakthroughs, developments, alerts, and vital information in medicine that I know are important to you, your family, and friends. The problem is that for the most part, only physicians learn of them—at our professional meetings and through the literature we read.
>   Therefore I've decided to do something about it. Every few months you'll receive from me these important ideas and concepts so you too can know and perhaps take needed action. So watch for them.
>   Now for your consideration, here are some of these important and even revolutionary developments.

In the letter, describe three or four enticing innovations in your field or your procedures. You might also remind patients of other services they may have forgotten. A multipage letter gives you the room to describe the benefits of a number of new developments and innovations, not just one. With more room, you can be more convincing. Don't worry about length. Just worry about maintaining interest.

The copy should create a sense of immediacy. Use "you," "your," and other personal pronouns to talk directly to the patient. Write short words, short sentences, and short paragraphs. Describe each development once, but mention its benefits over and over. Over and over and over. If the letters can be computer-generated and therefore personalized, take advantage of that ability. Tests have shown that the more times a person's name appears in the copy, the more readership you get.

Another Alternative—Other practices are using packaging suggestive of telegrams to reach their patients. Even those the addressee knows aren't true telegrams, like Trans-O-Gram, nonetheless, they feel these pieces of mail are official and demand immediate attention.

The inside message might begin as follows:

Dear _____,

We have just installed our new patient communications computer system. We now have a sophisticated tool to keep you abreast of the latest developments and innovation in _____ medicine.

One of those developments is . . .

The letter could summarize the latest developments and research in your field and explain the implications for your patients. That message demonstrates how up-to-date your own professional knowledge remains as well as educates your patients about preventive medicine and your own role in their health maintenance.

Here again the message is personalized. The copy also tells the patient that this practice is high-tech. And the patient is holding the proof in his or her hands. Moreover, either the letter or the format communicates that patients must read the next edition if they want to stay abreast of the latest developments. This copy has a *sense of excitement* that newsletters always lack.

An Example—Having learned the truth about newsletters, orthopedic surgeon R.T. took the better approach. He wrote a two-page letter touting three exciting developments in his practice. But more importantly, he explained what those advances really meant in his patients' lives. That information positioned the practice as *high-tech*, *highly advanced*, and *highly concerned*.

He also told his patients that with new technology in his office— and because his practice was one of the very few in the city to have it—the practice was becoming busier. Because he liked to reserve his most convenient times for his existing patients, he urged those patients interested in any of the new advances to call immediately.

New calls: Sixteen. Average income per patient: $438. Total revenue: $7,008. Now he was sure he was keeping his name in front of his patients. Conclusion: The *presentation* of the information (as well as what you say) makes the phone ring.

REFERENCES

1. Interview with Barbara Mehlman, copywriter, Ogilvy & Mather Inc, 2 East 48th St, New York, NY 10017.
2. Interview with Douglas Mueller, Gunning-Mueller Clear Writing Institute, 736 El Rodeo Rd, Santa Barbara, CA 93110.

■ PART 2   Your Tools

■ SECTION 2
Reaching Out To New Patients: A Tough
Problem With 20 Easy Solutions

■ CHAPTER 9
Public Relations And Publicity: Physicians' Biggest Mistakes And How To Correct Them

☐ THE LIMITS OF INTERNAL MARKETING

In a recent *Practice Builder* survey of marketing techniques, most practitioners said internal marketing was their sole method of promotion. Yet when asked if they had excess capacity, 83% of the strictly internal marketers said, "Yes."

Given their desire for fuller appointment books, they now have two choices: (1) to increase their internal efforts and (2) to promote to likely segments of the public. But when it comes to increasing their internal efforts, many practitioners already use fairly sophisticated internal tactics—a seven-step recall system, expansion by adding new services, regular patient contact, periodic promotions to existing patients, reinforcing referrers, incentives for staff marketing, and so forth. Still, these haven't been enough.

Why? Simply because there's only so much gold in "them thar hills." Dealing with a limited universe oftentimes doesn't produce enough to keep the practice humming at 100% capacity—even when you've maximized your efforts. Hence, the need to look beyond your own doors.

A practice can't afford to rely *only* on internal promotion. It's not uncommon for a practice to have 50% of its dollars coming in from new patients. Some practices have higher percentages, some lower. But practically all rely on "new" dollars to be profitable.

Priorities—Organize your internal efforts first. After all, it's easier to market to existing patients than those with whom you have no relationship. But if your internal effort is insufficient—and most of the time it is—then you must reach out and touch someone new.

☐ EIGHT GREAT WAYS TO GET PUBLICITY ON A SHOESTRING

Free publicity is the best publicity, not only because it doesn't cost you anything, but also because it's much more credible than paid advertising. For instance, one West Coast ophthalmologist performed eye surgery on a well-known actress. With her permission, he held a press conference to announce her condition. Within 30 days, coverage of that single announcement netted 27 inquiries and 11 new surgical cases. Quick and easy. But how can you accomplish the same? Jay Levinson suggests the several following ways in *Guerrilla Marketing*:[1]

Be Newsy—Even if you have the best media contacts, you still have to provide news to get a story or interview. If a martian lands on your roof, yes, you'll have made the news without trying. But usually you've got to generate news. So here are eight great ways to create news all by yourself.

1. Tie in with the news of the day. Issue statements in your professional capacity that pertain to news stories. Give opinions. Point out flaws. Raise major questions.
2. Stage an event—a health fair, a medical seminar for your prime prospects, a free screening or consultation for children, the elderly, or the poor.
3. Release useful information. In your professional readings, you'll come across an item that your community would be interested in. Include it in a press release. This is very easy to do.
4. Form a committee. Study a question related to your profession that has importance to your community. Choose a hot topic. And be the spokesperson for the group.
5. Give an award or scholarship. People love awards. Invent one that ties into your profession. Announce it each year with a ceremony and press coverage.
6. Make a prediction. If it's startling enough yet fairly likely to come true, it will be news and will enhance your reputation as an expert.
7. Celebrate your own business anniversary. Donate something to the community—free services, products, a special creation.
8. Do something incredible. Paint a mural on the outside of your building. Hold a press conference at an unusual spot—a loading dock to dramatize the rising incidence of back pain in adults.

Results—How well does this work? Georgia physician T.T. gave away Thanksgiving turkeys to new patients. But when 200 were left unclaimed on the giveaway day, he called the local minister to donate them to the poor. He turned his turkey promotion into a cornucopia by thinking to call the local media. He zoomed from an unknown to a local hero.

☐ EVALUATING PUBLIC RELATIONS: IS IT WORTH IT?

What is publicity worth? It's obviously difficult to answer this question with hard numbers, such as how many new patients did the publicity single-handedly generate. Public relations pros use total sales and cost of linage as the two most common measures of PR effectiveness.

Total Sales—Take your gross from the month the publicity occurred as well as the following month, and compare it to your gross for the same 2 months last year. The increase—or decrease—at least gives you a feel for whether your PR was effective. Of course, other variables that affect your gross were also different in the two periods. But if the changes in all the other variables were not overwhelming, most of the difference can be attributed to the publicity.

Cost of Linage—If the PR appeared in a newspaper or magazine, take the total number of lines written about you in that publication, and multiply it by the periodical's advertising rate. That gives you the cost of the space had you paid for it. If you appeared on radio or television, you can come up with a similar figure for the airtime devoted to you and what it would have cost you to pay for it. Repeat for all the media in which you received free publicity and total.

Comparing the two—sales and the would-be cost—makes it easy to figure if your publicity is a boom or bust.

☐ HOW TO BECOME AN EFFECTIVE SPEAKER

Plastic surgeon E.K. decided to promote his practice through free seminars targeted to women concerned about aging and to both male and female executives. He spend $8,600 for ads and media to promote the seminar and did so successfully. On that evening, 23 interested prospects attended.

But the good news stops here. E.K. was terrified. He trembled, had no voice inflection or modulation, and stumbled through his script. Even if his delivery had been inspiring, his copy was not. Written in textbook style, at best it was dry; at worst, incomprehensible. The bottom line: one new patient while the other 22 walked.

The Problem—Obviously, it was E.K. Even E.K. admitted that. He inspired no one at the seminar, although he's comfortable and effective one-on-one.

He realized that today's professionals need to reach out, to make an effective presentation, to convince, and they need to do so out in their community as well as in their offices—in seminars, at club meetings, on radio and television talk shows, at conventions, and the like. Opportunities abound, but he was the limiting factor.

The Solution—E.K. went to Toastmasters International to learn to become an effective speaker. Founded in 1924, it now boasts over 5,000 clubs worldwide and is the largest, oldest, and best nonprofit organization in the field.

Through their communication and leadership program as well as their club meetings, E.K. learned organized thinking and effective speaking. Specifically, he learned about breaking the ice, establishing his purpose, developing his points, clarifying meaning, being persuasive, making messages memorable, making speeches interesting and challenging, drawing pictures with his vocabulary, and mastering diction, dialect, and enunciation. Toastmasters put E.K. through his paces and then gave him practice and evaluation.

Results—After 6 months, E.K. was ready to hold his second seminar. This would be a gutsy move for most, but Toastmasters gave him the confidence to face the challenge. The bottom line: 19 attendees that he was able to translate into 9 new patients. (You can call your local Toastmasters International club, or contact the worldwide headquarters to find the club nearest you. The headquarters is located at 2200 N. Grade Ave., Santa Ana, CA 92711, or call [714] 542-6793).

☐ HOW TO GAIN SPEAKING ENGAGEMENTS

It's common knowledge that speaking engagements fill an appointment book. But how do you find out whom to approach? One way is to monitor the meetings column of the local newspaper. Before calling an association or a club, evaluate the business-getting potential of its meetings. If it fits your niche, call to introduce yourself, and suggest a topic you'd like to address.

☐ **Close Your Speeches Successfully**

At the close of a speech you're giving, round out all the ideas you've explored earlier. Refer again to the story, example, or illustration you used as the attention getter at the beginning of the talk. Or briefly restate your main thesis and purpose. *Don't* close with new information.

☐ **EXTRA MILEAGE FROM SPEECHES**

Most professionals know that giving speeches help fill their appointment books. But did you know there are ways to wring even more from the time you spend behind the podium? Bert Decker,[2] America's foremost authority on speech-giving, offers four ways to get extra mileage from each speech you give:

1. Convert your speech into an article for submission to professional publications. If accepted, mail a postcard to your patients informing them of its pending publication. Also put a notice in your practice newsletter. When the article is published, get reprints, and mail again to your patients. Repetition of your message is important, so tell them often how this respected publication looks to you for expertise. Why? Because no one leaves an expert.
2. Publish the speech in full, or excerpt it in your practice newsletter. Again, third parties who invited you to speak breed credibility.
3. Provide audio cassettes of your speech. Make them available to patients, and also have them on hand for listening in your waiting room.
4. Look for a newsworthy angle in the speech, and rewrite these points as a press release. You might find yourself on the front page or in front of the TV camera.

☐ **SEMINARS REAP BIG DOLLARS**

If you'd like your promotion to be low key, prestigious, and ethical, without raising any colleague's eyebrows, and have it reap big dollars, then take a lesson from Jamie Rower and Ira Bernstein, dentists in Suffern, NY.

For the past 3 years, these practitioners have been holding seminars to promote their practice. Result: 210 seminar attendees and 41 new patients. Better yet, most of those new patients had pressing cases of $1,000 or more each. That's over twice the practice's normal case size. Total gross: in excess of $50,000.

How To's—Doctors Rower and Bernstein target clubs and the public for their seminars. The clubs, of course, include the Lions and Rotarians. But response from women's groups turned out to be three times more favorable. So their targets have been changing—Women's Chapter of the Italian American League, Jewish women's groups, and so on.

How do they identify organizations? Both through their patients and by direct mail. And how do they publicize the event? Not only through the club's announcements, but also by doing their own mailing to the club members describing the seminar topic, cosmetic dentistry, and mentioning the length of the talk, 30 minutes.

These dynamic dentists have also held two seminars for the general public and have planned others. In their case, the local utility company provides the auditorium free of charge. Your local library is a possible spot at little or no cost. Publicity is accomplished through newspaper ads, some radio spots, and press releases to generate short announcements and to have the event mentioned in the local media's calendar listings. As a side benefit, that publicity may also succeed in generating patients directly because the public is impressed with professionals who lecture.

All promotion of these dentists has been in announcement format with the benefits buried in the copy. A better idea: Put the benefits in the headline.

During the Seminar—The two dentists have prepared 110 to 120 slides for their 30-minute show, about 3 slides per minute. They report that the question-and-answer periods are excellent. Good, tough, incisive questions are raised—the kind that make them shine.

During the seminar, they hand out literature as take-home material, plus a questionnaire that the attendees fill out at the end of the seminar to evaluate the presentation. In addition, they take attendees' names and addresses to add to their newsletter mailing list.

You Can Too—Seminars can pay big dollars for all professionals, except the most obscure specialists. But the topic is crucial. Choose it carefully for the greatest appeal. Then follow the formula.

☐ BOOSTING CREDIBILITY AND INCOME WITH SEMINARS

Whether a generalist is appealing directly to the public or a specialist to generalists for their referrals, seminars are a vehicle that can deliver two benefits—dollars and credibility. These free or minimum charge seminars are not only effective in producing patient flow, but they're looked on as low key, prestigious, and ethical.

But not everyone can give successful seminars. Some may not have enough presence to sound authoritative. But if it's a lack of nerve, don't worry. No seminar giver has ever been really ready to give his or her first one. But those who have given seminars recognize that if they had waited until they had felt confident, they would still be waiting today.

The Six Factors—Twenty-four seminar promoters recently gathered to discuss their marketing strategies.[3] The six factors they found most important for the success of a program are as follows:

1. *The topic itself*: Is there truly a need for the information from the point of view of your intended audience? And does the seminar title titillate? Of the six factors, a topic that's worthwhile and engrossing ranks as the second most vital ingredient. Construct a list of possible subjects. Ask people you know who belong to your target group which subject they'd find appealing. Consider testing two different seminar topics to find the optimal one.

2. *Price sensitivity*: Most professionals put seminars on for free, certainly when the target is other professionals. But sometimes practitioners are wise to charge a nominal fee. This reduces attendance, but those who do attend prove to be more interested and more qualified to buy your services.

3. *Location*: The image you want to convey is underscored by the meeting site. Beware of churches and schools. Churches may make people feel uncomfortable. And many schools are run down. A convenient location is also the key. If you're choosing a first-class hotel in your area, don't worry about the location. Their marketing research department confirmed its easy access before the place was built.

4. *Time of day, week, and month*: Should you schedule the seminar in the evening? A Saturday? A weekday? The answer comes from knowing your market. However, a survey of another 212 seminar givers ranked their most productive months in this order: January, September, October, April, March, June, November, February, December, May, July, and August.

5. *Length of Program*: One meeting or two? One, two, four or six hours? Again, the length comes from your market's needs.

And the most important variable?

6. *Promotion*: Success in seminars is more a function of marketing and promotion than program design, development, and instructional

competency. If you can't get them in the door, you can't dazzle them with your brilliance.

Promotion can be done a number of ways. Direct mail is often used *if* you can identify a mailing list of likely prospects. For specialists promoting to gain the referrals of general practitioners or allied professionals, this is a relatively easy task. The *Yellow Pages*, local professional association, state board, or a list broker will do the job easily. For other prospects, the task is harder, but not impossible. Just closely define your market. Look around for list sources. Consult a mailing list broker in the *Yellow Pages* under "mailing lists."

What to Mail—There are two alternative approaches to use here. First is the information intensive piece. It's not always the prettiest, but the formula is time-tested. Its components are bold headline, photos, strong benefit-oriented copy, testimonials, a section entitled, "What You Will Learn," your credentials, photos of any material to be provided, a reply mechanism for prospects to register for the seminar, an "act now" kicker, captions on all photos, and if appropriate, information on continuing education credit.

The other direct mail approach is an elegant invitation. It's printed on a card stock with appropriate wording to indicate that the prospect is cordially invited to attend a complimentary seminar on your designated topic. Include the address, time, and other particulars, as well as an R.S.V.P. with your phone number together with the phrase "limited seating" below it.

Which approach should you use? Testing is the only way to learn which one will work best.

Needle in the Haystack—But what if you can't identify the right mailing list to begin with? And mailing to everyone imaginable at 25 to 35 cents a piece is too costly to find the few prospects who need you? Then try newspapers or radio.

A successful newspaper ad follows the same copy guidelines as those for direct mail. Either the information intensive approach or the invitation can do well depending on your target and the subject you'll address. Schedule your newspaper ads to run at least on two Sundays preceding the seminar date. Preferably run additional weekday insertions as well.

Another alternative is the tickler ad designed to run frequently given its low cost. This is a 1-column × 1-in. ad with a large but terse headline: "SPORTS INJURY?" "BACK PAIN?" "NEARSIGHTED?" The two or three lines of copy describes the free or nominal-charge seminar, its purpose, and the phone number to call for more information. The phone is answered by a 60- to 90-second recorded announcement about the seminar. Callers then leave their name, address, and phone number to reserve a spot.

Use radio when your targets are younger people who don't read newspapers or for highly specific groups—the audience of a classical music station, which tends to be older and wealthier, or that of a psychological talk show. Remember: With radio, all your calls come in right after each spot airs, so have enough phone lines and personnel ready to handle them. For seminar reservations, using an answering service's multiple in-house lines, would be wise.

Other Tips—Forget posters. They tend to be the least productive form of seminar promotion. And again, don't be surprised if the seminar ads produce patients who don't attend the seminar. Some prospects will call wanting your services now.

If your seminar is for general practitioners from whom you wish to gain referrals, don't be afraid to share information with them for fear that they'll then turn around and do the procedure themselves. In the seminar, be clear and conversational when you run through the benefits of your expertise. But speak very technically, giving an abundance of difficult information that borders on being impossible to process. The generalists will conclude that it's too tough to handle, and therefore there's really only one person to refer to.

Follow up all attendees with a strong letter. Repetition works here also.

If appropriate, have someone from your staff sell materials at the back of the room. Those who don't want your services at the time may want books, cassettes, or other materials. Sales of $5 to $75 each add nicely to your monthly profits.

And most importantly, *don't* push your services. The hard sell loses. People look at it as a betrayal of trust. Instead, two or three times during the seminar, illustrate how your services have helped others. Your practice brochures and business card at each participant's seat will do the rest.

Results—Psychiatrist T.B. runs a $10 introductory seminar, "How to Be Happier in Any Relationship," to attract group therapy and individual patients. He draws an average of 18 attendees and typically attracts two new group therapy patients and one private patient per seminar. "This not only works, but it builds my reputation and helps my word-of-mouth referrals. There are also intangibles and spinoffs that you can't directly attribute to the seminars, but you suspect those seminars had something to do with it when after awhile you see the whole practice prosper."

☐ HOW TO GET ON RADIO/TV TALK SHOWS

For the professional looking for sophisticated, ethical, and altruistic promotion, put on your best suit, practice on your tape recorder, and become a guest on your local radio or TV talk show. A physician in Philadelphia appeared on a local TV show to discuss hypnotherapy and received an incredible 2,400 calls. Less impressive but certainly lucrative was the experience of a family practitioner in Seattle who received 119 calls after his appearance on a radio show. Publicist Ben Frank[4] suggests the game plan to put you on the air waves.

How to Get On—*Step 1*: Develop a topical idea—an "angle" in the trade. What's a subject of current interest that you can offer expertise on? What are people now questioning you about at dinner parties and other social occasions? Take issue with a current fad. If you can't think of an angle, consider a PR firm. That's what they do.

Step 2: Develop a press kit with subject summaries, your curriculum vitae, or resume, a list of other appearances, testimonials, reprints, and photos.

Step 3: Get on the phone. Call talk show producers and describe your angle and your qualifications. Your big problem: Busy producers are barraged by similar calls from agents, authors, politicians, and the like—persistence is a must. For success, cultivate the media, but don't pester them.

Once Is Not Enough—Don't stop the efforts once you've appeared as a guest. The public has a very short memory. To reinforce your

---

☐ A Round-Up of Sample Seminar Topics

1. Primary care physicians: "57 Ways to Stay Healthy and Live Longer."
2. Allergists: "How to Cure or Control Chronic Sinus Headaches, Hay Fever, and Asthma."
3. Cosmetic Surgeons: "The Newest Breakthroughs in Cosmetic Surgery: Now More Beautiful than Ever."
4. Obstetricians: "The 10 Most Important Steps During Your Pregnancy."
5. Ophthalmologists: "What Is Radial Keratotomy and How Does It Cure Nearsightedness?" or "Cataracts: What They Are and What You Can Do Today."
6. Orthopedic Surgeons: "The Back School: How to Take Care of a Bad Back," or "Sports Injuries: Getting Cured and Coming Back Strong."

☐ Free Media

If you're thinking of a special event to generate publicity and exposure, there's a way to guarantee free exposure and a healthy turnout.

Depending on your target market, contact either a local radio or television station, newspaper, or magazine to sponsor the public service event for its public relations value. The advantages for you: Free, repetitive advertising appealing to the publication or station's own audience; having the ads or spots produced without cost; and the benefit of gaining their expertise in marketing, again, at no cost.

The special events prime for media sponsorship: seminars; 10K runs and other athletic events; health fairs; exhibitions and community fairs.

---

image, continually cultivate your contacts. Then when news breaks and those contacts need a commentary, they'll think of you. Better yet, when your expertise bears on fast breaking news, seize the moment, and call the media yourself.

If this sounds like too much work, hire a public relations firm experienced in handling professionals. Then you'll pay someone else for their expertise, persistence, and time.

Results—Over a 2-year period, a public relations firm arranged 2 major newspaper articles, 30 local radio shows, and 10 local television appearances for surgeon R.Y. He notes, "Payoffs from PR don't always come right away, but our program has paid handsomely in the long run. My patient flow is well ahead of what it was before I started doing talk shows. As a matter of fact, one recent surgery case that came from these efforts alone paid for the entire program."

☐ HOW TO CREATE PUBLICITY WHEN NOTHING'S NEW

When there's absolutely nothing new in your practice, how can you maintain a high profile in your community? Here's one physician's answer.

When President Reagan's prostate surgery had just been disclosed and was fresh in the public's mind, internist W.H. launched a checkup program. He wrote to the top 100 company presidents in his area inviting them to come in for a free half-hour checkup and suggested that the CEO would be acting as a role model for that company's older workers thereby encouraging them to get regular checkups. He also pointed out that the early-detection regular checkups also helps keep health costs down.

As the acceptances began coming in, W.H. sent a press release to the local media as well as a publicity photo showing him with a patient. He also provided a story about the checkups to the employee newsletter of each company who's CEO had accepted.

Results—Thirteen CEOs accepted. Three of them became regular patients. Then 106 new patients came in from their companies over the next 60 days.

"If I hadn't done this," W.H. explains, "how else could I get so many well-qualified patients in here so quickly. This was the biggest boost to my practice . . . The way we did it also made me feel good."

Tactic—When you seize an event or issue important to your locale, tie the practice into it as tightly as possible. And do it quickly before the topic becomes old news. Avoid those tie-ins of dubious strength. Make sure there's a logical connection between your expertise and the event or issue. The more logical the connection, the stronger the conversion into new or renewed cases.

☐ IS A NEWSPAPER COLUMN REALLY WORTH IT?

The Practice Builder interviewed 15 professionals who had recently promoted their practices by providing their local newspaper with newspaper columns presented as a public service. Only one actually wrote the column that carried his byline. The other 14 purchased their columns from writing services. All had run their columns a minimum of 1 year, although nine have now discontinued them. Twelve of the 15 were required to pay the newspaper for running the columns.

The final accounting shows 12 of 15 reporting a few patients generated directly from their newspaper columns. Three reported a profitable experience, but none of the three paid for their columns' publication. All 15 felt the columns helped reinforce their image in their community.

If you're seriously considering buying or writing your own newspaper column, enter the program with few expectations and armed with a strategy to keep the costs down.

Cost Containment—First, you shouldn't pay for the space in which to run your column. Approach editors of your local paper or magazine with the offer of providing a public service which will increase their readership and bind their existing readers to the publication. Approach those publications with the greatest readership in your office's area first. Work your way down the readership ladder from there.

You'll find that new local magazines or newspapers will be your most receptive audience. Be the first one there, and come with a good sample of your column.

Avoid investing continual sums to appear in a format that may not pay back that investment. But that caution can be tempered with two exceptions. If your name would appear without cost, welcome the gift horse, and use the columns to build your name recognition for the long term. Likewise, if you enjoy writing for its own sake, that too changes the picture. Otherwise, newspaper columns rarely add to your bottom line.

☐ RADIO EDITORIALS

Why have studies found that newspaper columns presented as a public service generate little response? Perhaps the reason is that newspaper readership is weak for those under 40 years of age or that readership is on the decline.

What is working now are those same editorials—delivered on radio. Depending on the station, they reach younger people as well as older. And there's another difference. With newspapers, each reader must first decide to look at the paper. Then the person must choose to read that particular article or ad. But radio is an *intrusive media:* Listeners need only decide to listen to your station. So actual delivery to the audience is much higher than with newspapers and other print media.

Format—The radio spots are hard to distinguish as advertising. An announcer introduces the 60-second spot as "Ask the Doctor." The announcer then asks a question of common interest that permits you to display your acumen and poise. The end of the spot can suggest that for more information or an appointment, call Dr. _____ . The phone number is repeated at least twice.

And the impression? That the station looks to you as the area's resident expert in your field. Why else would they have you as a regular feature.

As one doctor explained, "I ran for 6 months on a local station, increased my gross about 20%, and not one patient knew that I paid for that air time."

☐ DIAL-A-DOCTOR: CALL-IN RADIO

The physician sits down behind his desk, flips a few switches, makes a phone call, and begins talking to hundreds of people on his "Dial-A-Doctor" call-in radio program. He's part of the rush into broadcasting that have found professionals of every stripe taking their advice to the airwaves in radio markets across the country.

What's interesting about these public relations programs is that few of the professionals had ever before thought of themselves as would-be media personalities. None of them had experience. And all but a few *buy* the time for their shows from the radio station.

Pros and Cons—Advantages: It's a low-key, high-profile, public-service approach to promotion that doesn't involve "selling." All you do is dazzle your audience with your knowledge. Disadvantages: It's time consuming—many practitioners broadcast an hour a day, 5 days a week.

The other disadvantage is the cost. It varies by size of market, the station's market share, and whether you do everything yourself or hire a consultant. Hiring a consultant ups the tab to about $3,000 to $8,000 per month, again, depending on the market. Doing everything yourself lops off half that cost or more.

How To—First pick the radio station. Look for those that cover your geographical market area without exceeding it too much. Then look for those with listener demographics that match those of your patients and prospects. (Interestingly, all-talk formats and Christian stations often have among the most responsive audiences.)

When you find the right station, open negotiations. The station's concern will be the risk of losing listeners with a show by an untrained broadcaster. Your object is to convince them that they won't. Then negotiate the radio costs.

Special telephone equipment will need to be installed in your office to link it with the station to ensure that callers are heard clearly and an overall good quality feed. Look to the station for details.

Once you've started broadcasting, don't solicit business on the show. This is accomplished with commercials about your practice played several times during the show. Those commercials should be taped by a professional announcer who talks about the practice to maintain your noncommercial credibility.

Thrifty Idea—In larger radio markets, two physicians who serve different parts of the same market can joint venture the program. It's half the work, half the cost, and about the same results.

And the results? The picture's mixed. One practitioner who took to the airwaves reported 318 new patients in 6 months, but another landed only 2 new patients per program, while yet another quit after 3 weeks of no results.

Several factors differentiate the winners from the losers:

1. The practitioner must want to do the program. If there's any reluctance, it will come across, and the show will be boring.

2. Choosing the right station and time slot will make or break the effort. Be careful.

3. Don't think short term. Long term seems to pay. Expectations of overnight success means failure.

4. Learn from criticism. Without proper broadcast training, you have a long way to go to become another Dr. Art Ulene or Toni Grant.

Professional Help—A few marketing people are turning to this area to offer their expertise. Some have a ready-made package for professionals that includes finding the station, negotiating the arrangement, installing the equipment, then training you and your staff, and finally producing the commercials about your practice that will air during your program.

If it seems like work, it is. The start-up stage is time consuming, the choices critical. But once you're underway, the regimen is smooth.

REFERENCES

1. Levinson J: *Guerrilla Marketing*, Boston, Houghton Mifflin Co, 1984, p 87.
2. Decker B: Communicating par excellance. *Decker Communications Report*, February 1986, p 4, 607 N Sherman Ave, Madison, WI 53703.
3. Shenson HL: *How to Develop And Promote Profitable and Successful Seminars and Workshops*. Woodland Hills, Calif, Howard L. Shenson, 1985.
4. Interview with Ben Frank, Ben Frank Promotion Corp, 60 E 42nd St, New York, NY 10017.

■ CHAPTER 10
Professional Referrals And Marketing Within PPOs, IPAs, HMOs: Learning To Use Today's Newest Strategy

☐ NEW METHOD BOOSTS PROFESSIONAL REFERRALS 20%

How do you convince practitioners in allied fields that you deserve their referrals? Louisiana physician M.J. found one way.

After seeing a new patient, M.J. sends a letter to the personal dentist whom the patient listed on his chart. The doctor reports on the patient's health and explains that he hopes the information might be of assistance in assessing the patient's dental health. He writes not only to the patient's dentist, but to all the health professionals that patient uses. It's all done with the patient's permission and then generated by computer.

Such a letter would show your concern and reflects on the thorough care you deliver. Of course, it never asks for referrals. Its purpose is strictly to increase your name recognition and enhance your professional image. M.J. does, however, include his practice brochure with the letters he sends. Of the 60 new patients M.J. saw the month after he'd begun the program, 12 had come from professional referrers who had been sent the letter and brochure.

Strategic Applications—Write to the appropriate specialists or generalists and to allied practitioners in different professions: For instance, general practitioners to dentists, chiropractors, podiatrists, ophthalmologists, and so on. Of course, check local regulations for disclosure restrictions.

As with most promotions, the more often you communicate with the other professionals, the more likely you'll receive referrals because the more they'll view you as thorough, caring, and an expert. These extra steps alone are enough to differentiate you from a sea of competing practitioners.

☐ AND ANOTHER WAY TO BOOST YOUR REFERRALS

A more direct approach is that taken by psychiatrist M.R. He sent 300 letters to nearby physicians to solicit referrals. The letter focused on his credentials and pointed out his specialty of treating alcohol and other drug abuse. But the results were poor: one referral from one doctor in 6 months.

A Vote of No-Confidence—Professionals only refer to colleagues they know and feel comfortable with and to those they recognize as experts. Why? Because the recommendation reflects back upon the referring practitioner's own stature and credibility with his or her patients. M.R.'s letter may have made a start in winning the confidence needed for a referral but fell woefully short of completing the process. Therefore, for increased referrals, first position yourself as an expert. And then introduce yourself to potential referrers.

But how does one become an expert? Simply by having people call you one. So the productivity of this strategy centers on establishing a forum for you to prove your expertise. Then you must publicize how third parties acknowledge you as an authority in your field.

Tactics—First create your forum—a quarterly newsletter for physicians and allied health professionals in which you can act as an oracle of your profession or specialty. Your newsletter should contain information about your field that those sophisticated readers would find useful and interesting. Include case histories that illustrate how to recognize when to refer a patient to another practitioner such as yourself. Include other information from the literature that those readers might apply in their daily work. The more useful the articles, the more the newsletter will be read. An example of such a newsletter is shown in Figure 10–1.

Secondly, compile a mailing list of all potential referrers in your area. Don't overlook professionals in other fields such as the clergy, social workers, or psychologists who come in contact with your prospective patients.

Key Concept—The newsletter puts you in print, automatically establishing your credibility. The newsletter marks you as the authority to turn to in your field. Keep in mind several guidelines. To get your newsletter read, write about people. Make your point from the case

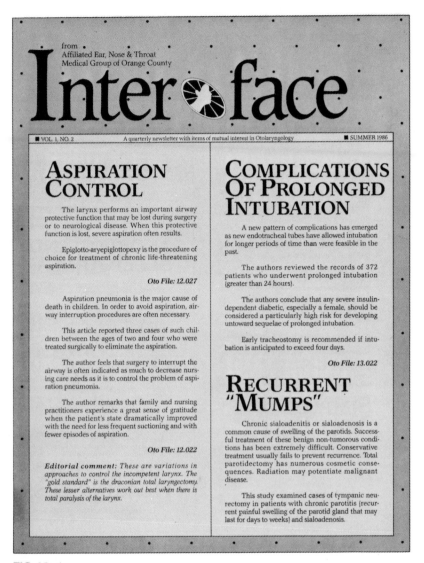

FIG 10–1.

histories. Otherwise, your writing will tend to sound academic and boring.

Also include a section on your upcoming talks, classes, radio or television appearances, as well as newspaper, magazine, or journal articles. What appears here is any invitation, solicited or otherwise, from any organization, club, or media. These presentations and articles are evidence that you're seen as an expert.

Production—Format the newsletter as a four-pager (an 11×17-in. sheet folded in half to a finished size of $8 \, ^1/_2 \times 11$ in.). Have a commercial artist design a masthead and a layout master into which you'll drop each issue's finished copy. Cost: about $200 to $300. Write and type your articles to the size of the format. Each month have the artist lay out the articles on the master layout and set the headlines. Cost: $50 to $100. Give it to your local quick printer. Mail the first issue first class. Bulk mail subsequent issues at about half the postage if you send out quantities of 200 or more copies.

Write a cover letter to be included with that first issue explaining how you've noticed that carefully selected information from your field is needed in practices like that of the reader and how you hope this complimentary newsletter will fill that void, providing helpful items important to the reader's practice and his or her patients.

Also point out that you're available to answer questions about any of the newsletter's articles or how they apply to the reader's practice. In addition, tell him or her you're more than happy to provide your professional opinion on any case. The reader should feel free to call.

Then list your credentials for the reader's information. Emphasize experience, training, areas of expertise, articles, or talks you've given, professional association memberships and positions. Don't hold back.

Follow-Up—With your credibility established, you're now ready to introduce yourself to fulfill all the requirements for ongoing referrals.

Start calling the practitioners on your mailing list. Ask if they've received the newsletter and if they have any questions about the articles. Reiterate that you're also happy to provide opinions about cases or issues so they should feel free to call. If the conversation moves well, offer to meet for lunch or to arrange an office meeting.

Repetition of contact is once again the key to success. If the first series of follow-up calls net X referrals, the second will produce four times that, and the third even more. Subsequent follow-ups always produce more than earlier ones.

More Contact—Each time you schedule a class, talk, media appearance, or article, send a postcard to your mailing list beforehand:

> Dear Colleague,
> On Saturday, April 4, at 6 A.M., I'll be speaking on WKRP about (topic). I invite you to listen because I know this information is important to you and your patients.

Not that anyone will necessarily get up at 6 A.M. that Saturday, but now they'll know that, again, someone else considers you an authority. And after the appearance, do another mailing offering a synopsis of the talk or a copy of the article. Why? Because repetition works. Repetition works. Repetition works.

Results—M.R. implemented the program exactly as written, mailing and contacting his list of 300. After the first go-through, he reduced the list to 165 prime prospects for phoning, but continued to mail to all 300. In 6 months of concerted effort, he received 118 direct referrals and added two associates. "The start-up took awhile, but after the second follow-up, all the efforts paid handsomely. Now I don't need to do any other kind of promotion . . . . Is it work? Certainly. Does it pay? Definitely."

☐ CLOSED GROUP MARKETING TO BUSINESS

Friends from three different professions had an idea. They knew that businesses are worried about containing the cost of employee

---

☐ Savvy Tactic: The Co-op Referral List

Is there a way to substantially increase the referrals from those practitioners who already refer to you? This was the question one G.P. asked and who then came up with a savvy technique.

He contacted all the professionals to whom he normally referred or recommended patients and offered to place their names on his soon-to-be publicized referral list. The list would be placed in his waiting room for all his patients to see as well as publicized in his newsletter. In addition to including the specialists to whom he referred, he also contacted practitioners such as a pedodontist and an optometrist whom he trusted and therefore would recommend if a patient were to ask.

Reciprocal Arrangement—He recommended that all of the other practitioners he contacted adopt this time-saving way to communicate with their own patients by providing their own list of the practitioners they recommended. Of course, his name was shown on those lists.

"The reason it works so well," he explains, "is that instead of a colleague telling only a handful of patients about me, almost all of his current patients have seen the listing that shows me as one of the recommended general practitioners. Eight different professionals have agreed to publicize their referral list with me on it. I've now received 6 new patients from 1 office alone and a total of 21 newly referred patients this last month."

Suggestion—Stick to closely related professions. The closer the relationship, the greater the credibility of the referral. And the greater the in-house promotion, the more business generated.

---

benefits but are still pressured by their employees to expand their benefits packages. The three practitioners said, "Why don't we discount our services to them—much like a PPO or IPA does—in exchange for a healthy ongoing volume of patients. If a company is willing to make this part of its benefit package and promote it, then the plan should work."

The company would benefit since the plan would extend their package by working with their existing insurance plans and by extending coverage into areas previously not covered—all at no cost.

The employees would benefit from those additional goodies that they would receive at a reduced cost. And the practitioners would benefit from the increased patient flow. The three professionals realized, "It fits our needs, it fits the company's needs, and it fits the employee's needs—a perfect WIN-WIN-WIN situation."

In this case, the group decided to include a broad range of professionals in the plan, but the concept could be executed for a single profession as well. They also decided to market their services as a package to businesses. Why as a package? Because a number of them had tried by themselves to gain access into businesses near their front doors only to fail. They ran into objections, many of them, but as a group, they felt they could answer them all.

Common Objectives—Typical were the objections given to W.R. when he alone approached three large corporations within a mile of his office. First, he was told that there were so many employees that W.R. couldn't possibly handle them all. So limited capacity took him out of the game (unless the businesses were small or his service so specialized or unique that demand would be limited).

The companies also told him that with the proposed plan covering employees and their families who live all over the county, his office was inconvenient for many would-be participants.

The third objection, which they didn't tell him, is that if the company did this with W.R., they'd have a whole stream of other individual practitioners wanting to do the same thing—and who's got time for all that? Besides, we're talking to someone from the personnel department who likes rules and the status quo, not innovation or anything out of the ordinary.

The Group Solution—A group of noncompeting practitioners could overcome all these objections. With a variety of dispersed offices, convenience was no longer a problem. With multiple offices, neither was capacity. And with a group, the unimaginative clerk in personnel wouldn't have to deal with screening individual practitioners.

Then the three decided to enhance their package. To begin with, they could charge 75% of their usual and customary fees, unless insurance paid more—in which case they would accept the assignment as payment in full. This was a highly attractive savings so employees would utilize the plan. For each participating practitioner, this was income in addition to his or her normal work load. What with overhead already paid for by existing patients, the new income was all profit except for the cost of additional materials used. (That's known in economics as the theory of marginal profit.)

Then to put at rest employees' fears that prices had first been raised before they were discounted 25%, the standard fee schedule was available at each practitioner's front desk.

Other practitioners interested in participating were prescreened in five different ways to assure quality control in the program. Backgrounds were checked, offices inspected, and only experienced professionals permitted to join. The plan certainly appealed here, too. More than 100 practitioners were chosen to offer a myriad of disciplines. It even included veterinarians, lawyers, accountants—an unusual spectrum of professional services discounted for the employees.

The plan was easy to use. All the employee had to do was call the central referral number for the practitioners in his or her area. In this way, no hard-to-find directories were needed, and lists could be updated at a moment's notice. The large costs of directory printing were also avoided.

Lastly, they packaged the plan as a nonprofit corporation to give it that extra bit of credibility—not only for employees but also for the businesses.

Whom to Approach and How—Not all businesses are prime for this idea. Large, self-insured corporations with more than 200 or 300 employees usually see this approach as increasing utilization and therefore costing them more.

So prime targets are organizations that are not self-insured. For these, first approach them by direct mail. A cover letter with the brochure (Fig 10–2) was sent to the five most likely decision makers in each organization. Multiple pieces were mailed to each organization because an outsider can rarely pinpoint the appropriate decision makers with any accuracy. The rule: It's better to overmail than undermail.

The one-color brochure shown in Figure 10–2 is dramatic. The headline is dramatic. The visuals are captivating. And the copy is compelling. Notice the use of subheads to break up thoughts into easily digestible chunks; also how the copy moves quickly with short words, short sentences, and short paragraphs; and how the graphic symbols give substance to the words. Printed in black on card stock, this is actually an inexpensive printing job. Only the design and writing were costly.

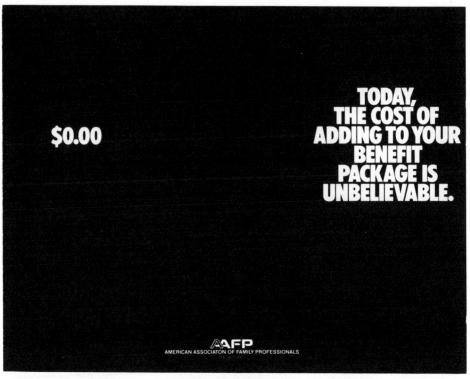

At a time when high rates are forcing some organizations to reduce benefits, the American Association of Family Professionals is reducing costs.

The AAFP Benefit Plan is a new concept that allows its members to receive a 25% fee reduction on more than 30 professional services.

dontists, and family practitioners.

In case you can't see in the chart, vision care is also included. Along with veterinarians.

And all AAFP member professionals charge 25% less than non-member professionals. Enrollees will even be allowed to compare AAFP practitioners' fee

Accountants	Physicians	Psychiatrists
Acupuncturists	Allergists	Rheumatologists
Attorneys	Dermatologists	Urologists
Chiropractors	Ear, Nose &	Other Specialists
Dentists	Throat	**Podiatrists**
General	Specialists	**Psychological**
Practitioners	Family &	**Counselors**
Oral Surgeons	General	Licensed Clinical
Orthodontists	Practitioners	Social Workers
Pedodontists	Gynecologists	Licensed
Endodontists	Internists	Psychologists
Periodontists	Obstetricians	Marriage, Family
Specialists	Ophthalmologists	& Child
Optometrists	Orthopedic	Counselors
Osteopathic	Surgeons	**Registered**
Physicians	Pediatricians	**Dieticians**
Physical	Plastic Surgeons	**Veterinarians**
Therapists		

And it won't cost you one red cent. Which will help keep your budget in the black.

We cover everything from A to V.

Even though AAFP can give your people healthy cost reductions, it isn't limited to just health care.

As you can see in the chart, accounting services are covered as thoroughly as allergists, gynecologists, ortho-

structures to those of non-members. So there's no question they'll be receiving everything you didn't pay for.

Of course, AAFP is not designed to replace the insurance or other benefits you currently offer. It merely enhances your package by extending coverage further than any of your insurance programs possibly could.

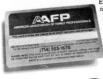

Needless to say, your people will put a premium on a benefit like that. But we won't.

Our bottom line is quality.

AAFP is a non-profit professional association with a membership numbering in the hundreds. And hundreds of organizations like yours are currently taking advantage of our services. Representing industries as diverse as pharmaceuticals, electronics, engineering, office equipment, manufacturing and food service.

Why have we been so successful? Because of what we make every member professional pay: Careful attention to the quality of their service.

Every doctor, attorney, counselor and, yes, even veterinarians are thoroughly prescreened in five ways. First, we check with the State Licensing Board. Then the member's Local Professional Association and the Better Business Bureau. We examine any history of malpractice. And finally, we make a personal office visit to make sure their premises meet the high standards of the association.

We also insist that our member professionals have an established practice. No recent graduates are permitted to join. And we limit our members to sole practitioners or small partnerships. So enrollees will never have to put up with noisy, crowded clinics.

We're easy to take advantage of.

Anyone who has a finger can use our services. All they have to do is phone AAFP (Monday-Friday, 8:30 to 5:30) to request the name of the nearest AAFP member in the category of service they require. We'll usually give them at least two choices. Often times, more. And since we have so many practicing members, they are almost always convenient to an enrollee's office or home. Now, if you've been reading this entire brochure waiting for the catch, you can stop waiting. There isn't any. All you do is inform your people of the

AAFP plan. At your convenience, one of our representatives will meet with you to thoroughly explain how our program works and to help you implement the plan. We'll also give you membership cards, fliers, posters and newsletter articles to keep enrollees informed about AAFP. At your request, we can even provide speakers.

Of course, there are a few things we won't give you. Like paperwork, procedures and complaints. Nor will there be a contract or any charges to your organization at any point. So you'll be able to incorporate the AAFP program without budgetary or home office approval.

Call us at (714) 851-9977. We'll show you how unbelievably easy it is to increase your benefit package with AAFP.

In fact, there's really nothing to it.

FIG 10–2.

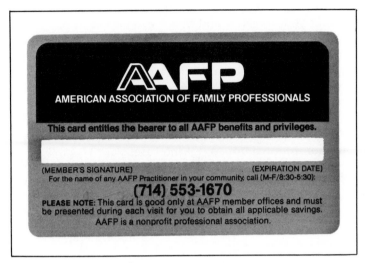

FIG 10–3.

Remember: If the piece is not first-rate, corporations will have nothing to do with you. Caveat: Invest in design and writing to avoid any hint of the second-rate or amateurish.

Follow up with a phone call. Then face-to-face meetings are needed to close the arrangement. And what was the arrangement? The organization could have the package at no cost if they would include it in their benefit package and allow the group to promote use of the package to employees. With no cost to the company, there were no budgeting problems. And no contracts, so no home office approval was required either, which would have bogged down everything.

The Key to Success—Corporate acceptance of the program doesn't mean success. Those unimaginative people haunting the halls of personnel will simply mention the plan in the back of the benefits book and forget about it. Promoting it or even informing employees about it in a meaningful way usually requires too much creativity.

But promotion is the key. Repetition, as in any other arena, works here, too. Since personnel won't or can't do it, you must. Here are six vital pieces to the successful promotional program:

1. *Membership card*: Made out of thin plastic, the card displays the phone number to call for referrals as seen in Figure 10–3. Each member of the family gets one so everyone can carry the plan in their pocket.

2. *Paycheck stuffer*: This is actually the main explanatory brochure for the user. But create it in the shape and size of a paycheck so it can be included in their pay envelopes on payday. Why? Because

when a company encloses something with your check, you know they want you to read it and that they endorse it.

3. *Telephone stickers:* Hand out at least two for each employee—one for home, one for work. Along with the referral number, list emergency numbers to enhance usage of the stickers and therefore the plan as seen in Figure 10–4. At 1 or 2 cents, these are very inexpensive promotional vehicles.

4. *Newsletter articles:* If the company has a newsletter, offer to write a monthly, quarterly, or occasional column. They're always looking for information. And it increases your visibility.

5. *Speaking engagements:* Also ranking high on visibility is speaking. Prepare a 20-minute talk plus questions and answers for a perfect 30-minute lunchtime or between-shifts appearance. After all, face-to-face is the most influential of all types of communication.

6. *Posters:* Reminders in the lunchroom, locker room, and hallways help build repetition as seen in the poster shown in Figure 10–5. Remember to keep your marketing themes and graphic look consistent to assist recognition.

Results—With over 100 practitioners pooling their moneys to pay for the promotional materials and the staff to promote the plan to organizations, it resulted in a bonanza: over 20,000 employees and their families covered in just 6 months' time.

"Since it was designed as a WIN-WIN-WIN program, everyone won," explained one of the organizers. "Well, almost everyone. We did have some practitioners who didn't do well on the program; we think it was mostly due to their office locations on the outskirts of the area we serve. So we're being more careful how we locate our professionals."

☐ MARKETING BY COHABITATION

Ever think you could increase your practice load simply by living with someone? Professionally, that is. Family physician B.C. discov-

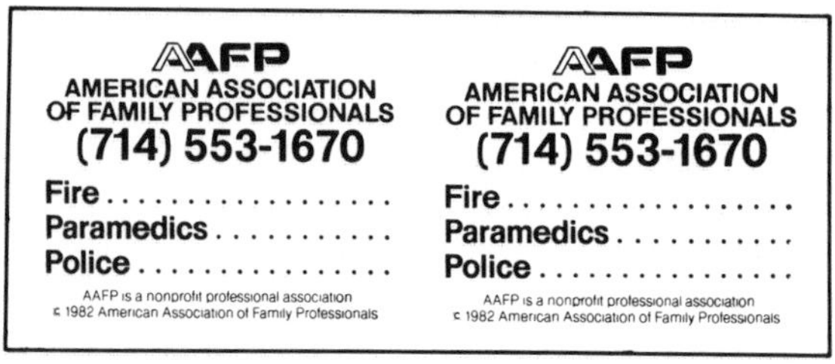

FIG 10–4.

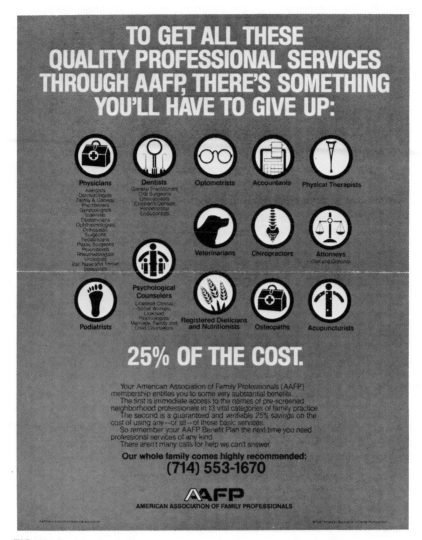

FIG 10–5.

ered exactly that when he wanted to move into a larger office and asked his friend and general dentist T.L. to share the space.

B.C. argued that the advantages were overwhelming:

1. They could both afford a better location and a larger, more spacious, better decorated office at less cost than they could individually.

2. Not only could rent be shared, but also other overhead items like the waiting room, receptionist, copier, and phone system would be divided between them.

3. The camaraderie of a noncompeting professional and friend in the office would be welcomed, and each would feel less isolated than practicing alone, but yet each would have the independence of running his own practice.

Thus, that list of advantages are the same pluses that justify sharing office space with a colleague in the same field. What surprised B.C. and T.L. were the profitable hidden advantages of the arrangement.

Cross Marketing—They found that the goodwill each of them had with his own patients transferred by association to the other. Simply by sharing a waiting room with a common receptionist, the patients of one practitioner began using the services of the other—something you wouldn't find when two practitioners in the same discipline share space.

The convenience of coming to the same office was another advantage since people began booking back-to-back appointments to see the two professionals. Another plus: The fact that the waiting room was always filled gave the impression of a successful practice. And people only want to go to successful professionals.

The results were a dramatic boost of over 20% in each professional's volume.

More Cross Marketing—The arrangement worked so well that they took their marketing a couple of steps further. First, business cards for both were available throughout the waiting room to better market to each other's patients.

Second, each wrote a series of letters announcing their move and the benefits of it to their patients. And in the letters, they announced the services of the other practitioner. Then after awhile, they began a cooperative monthly flyer called *The Medical-Dental Update* for both patient bases. It gave them a more consistent exposure in their patients' minds than they had had with their individual quarterly newsletters.

Cohabitation Guidelines—What makes sense is joining forces between professions with noncompeting but complementary services— for example, pediatrician and pedodontist, or ophthalmologist and OB/GYN. But beware: To succeed, each practitioner *must* have the same primary target market in terms of age, socioeconomic level, and perhaps sex. There's no synergism between an internist's patients 55 years or older and an orthodontist's youngsters and their mothers. It's a mix of oil and water. When the two patient bases mix well, the cross marketing will be a synergistic success.

☐ CASE HISTORY: CO-OP PROMOTION

Recently, a local southeast pediatric society invited *The Practice Builder* for a consultation about a very threatening problem—the loss of patients to quickly growing, free-standing emergency centers.

In this case, the competition was from clinics. But it could have been from HMOs, mobile clinics, franchises, or more likely from too many practitioners nearby. Although the details and some strategies will change, the answer—the basic co-op concept—can work in each case. It's applicable to professionals in general medicine or any specialty.

Time to Act Is Now—With eight emergency centers popping up in just 1 year, the pediatricians were justifiably concerned over losing their bread-and-butter business to these easy-access centers with extended hours.

But there's another reason the pediatricians' fears are well founded. As now positioned, these emergency centers primarily compete with area hospital emergency rooms that also treat trauma. But as their learning curve grows, emergency centers will soon realize they can deliver multispecialty, one-stop medicine. The trauma treatment will be just one service of many, all of which will be available at hours convenient to families in which both parents work—70% of households today.

This kind of repositioning will give the emergency centers repeat business to fully utilize their assets. And that is when the pediatricians (as well as other primary care practitioners) will really feel the brunt of competition. Before that happens, act now.

The Strategy—Compete with the centers on the basis of quality of care. Board certified-eligible in pediatrics means extensive training and an expertise that the emergency centers can't match. To parents, that means a more accurate diagnosis, more appropriate treatment, and an environment created to make a child feel comfortable, which also translates in a parent's mind into better care. When explained this way, would a mother rather take her child to the cold, frightening environment of a trauma center that has more experience in cardiac arrests than ear infections?

The Big Problem—To combat the large media budget of an emergency center and to convince parents to forego the center's convenient hours take repetition of the message. Prospects aren't likely to respond the first or second time they hear, see, or read what board certification means to them. The average person requires five to seven repetitions of a message before he or she is comfortable and motivated enough to act.

Public relations such as articles, speeches, and other appearances carry the implied endorsement of the media or organizations sponsoring the appearance. But the frequency of the endorsement falls short of the repetition needed for large-scale results.

The ideal combination to spread the word is public relations plus advertising. Yet given the repetition needed, the average sole practitioner can't afford the cost of the advertising portion of the equation.

The Big Solution—Promote cooperatively. Create a media pool, not under the banner of the pediatric society, but under a new organization created for that purpose. The pool need not include all society members. It could just be a small group of pediatricians who would also then compete against the stodgier members.

This pool solves the affordability problem. You can now divide media bills so you actually reach more people for less out-of-pocket costs than if flying solo. Plus, you can now afford major media—the big newspapers, the regional buys of the big national magazines, and the big broadcast stations. They deliver your message to more people at less cost per person than the very localized media you could afford on your own. And this is the key—the economies of scale and the power of co-op buying.

For the Really Big Payback—Not only overwhelm the competition with your superior training and credentials, but demolish them by offering extended hours to take away their competitive edge. Combine this double-barrel approach with total saturation co-op advertising, and the emergency centers will cause this professional group no more trouble.

To give the repetition time to produce and to fine tune the program, have all participants commit to a 6-month test. Use contracts and promissory notes to firm the commitments and to avoid having some members change their minds 2 weeks after the start. Agreement in writing also preserves friendships. Every month participants then pay into the pool.

For coordination of the campaign, hire a local ad agency and charge it with the creative process, media selection, and timing and production. Appoint only a three-person committee to oversee the agency—a larger committee will compromise everything to total blandness. Also charge the committee with coordinating the public relations efforts—speeches, articles, and broadcast appearances.

To assure that media pool members receive the patients gener-

ated, set up a central telephone referral number. Lease existing telephone lines on a rotary series from an answering service set up to
receive large numbers of calls at one time from advertising. Have
operators provide two or three names of the members nearest the
caller. Also have operators take names and daytime phone numbers
for forwarding to the recommended practitioners. If equipment permits, patch the call directly through to the office selected for one-step
appointment scheduling.

What to Expect—Usual returns range from four to five times the cost
to up to ten times. But that is just the start. Residuals include repeat
business in the future plus referrals. This makes each new pediatric
patient actually worth over $13,000 in the long run. And it doesn't

---

☐ Why Professional Associations Shouldn't Promote

Contrary to the title of this section, professional associations really should
promote the services of their members to the public. They're in an ideal position
to do so. They're big enough to pool members' moneys and to buy efficient
media in a large enough quantity to make a promotional campaign really zip
along. And they already have the organizational structure in place.

They're a perfect vehicle for accomplishing the job. Unfortunately, they're
incapable of doing the job.

The Nature of the Beast.—Being political creatures, medical societies and
other professional associations thrive on involving their members in decision
making. The result is a series of committees with everyone saying, "I think . . . "
and no one with a marketing background and the authority to say, "I know . . . ."
Consequently, emotions carry the day instead of a strategic marketing plan that
maximizes on a calculated analysis of the marketplace.

In those rare instances when an association adopts a promotional plan,
chances are the members will restrict the dues surcharge to a minimum, arguing
that they want to first see if the plan produces. They'll agree to commit more
funds *if* it works on a test.

Unfortunately, that's backwards. To show acceptable results, expenditures
need to be front-loaded. Then the plan can build the repetition of message
necessary to generate appointments. Without the dollars up front, the plan is
doomed.

Form Your Own.—Even with associations that appear on the surface to
be the perfect vehicle for promoting a profession or specialty, while many have
tried, none can or have succeeded.

So instead of waiting around for the exception, form your own promotional
group. Then you'll avoid the pitfalls of the political association filled with members who don't want to promote while still gaining the advantage of high dollar-
buying power.

just apply to pediatrics. No matter what the specialty, cooperative promotion delivers big pluses.

☐ EVALUATING CO-OP VENTURES

Promotional co-ops are becoming much more common for good reason. When set up properly, the results can be astonishing—perhaps 30 or 40 times return on investment. But the losses can be big, too. Here's a checklist to make sure your co-op produces only smiles.

1. *Territories*: Make sure all participating physicians are noncompeting. In urban areas this could mean an exclusive territory as small as 1 to 2 miles in radius; in suburbia, 3 to 5 miles; in rural markets, even more. The doctors located in the middle of the media market will receive far more respondents. To compensate the other participants, make their outlying territories larger.

2. *Media coverage*: Whether radio, TV, newspaper, or magazine, check if the proposed media delivers to your prime prospects *in your territory*. It may deliver for others in your co-op, but not for you. If so, beware! And consider co-op ventures where all the members are in your local media market. National co-ops don't have enough members or bucks to cover your market well.

3. *Expertise*: There are experts and there are "experts." Look at the track record of the creative and media people who are to handle the co-op's account. Do they know the optimal strategy for promoting your specialty? And do they know how to differentiate you as a group from competitors? Or is their expertise in restaurants and racquetball clubs? Don't let an "expert" learn on your money.

4. *Commitment*: The greatest problem in running a group is getting 5 to 50 doctors walking in lockstep in the same direction at the same time. That's exactly what a program like this requires. A co-op won't work without cooperation, and the only way to get it is to use 6-month contracts backed up by promissory notes. Any shorter duration doesn't give the advertising a fair chance to succeed because of the repetition needed. The promissory notes are needed to assure funding for the program. All notes should be prepaid *before* the media is run. The participating doctors are *not* to pay that month's media bills out of receipts. Prepayment also avoids the problem of cold feet and nonfunding due to lack of short-term results. All three keys are necessary: the 6-month commitment, contracts, and notes.

5. *Steering committee*: Advertising can't be produced or evaluated by a large committee, talented or otherwise. What comes out of a committee is bland creativity and compromised effectiveness. Yet while

everyone shouldn't vote on everything, the advertising people need to be steered. Choose three talented members with one as chief. No more. Not if you want effective promotion.

6. *A strong leader:* Pick a chief who has what it takes to be a strong leader. Doctors who part with money become nervous waiting for the payoff. (Who doesn't?) The leader's job is to do some hand holding with the participants until the program produces significant results. This is the hardest part for any chief. Without the leader assuming this role, there will be no group 4 weeks after the campaign breaks.

7. *Sufficient budget*: There must be enough media bucks to make a dent in the market. However, the usual tendency is to cut members' costs to the bone to attract more recruits to the co-op. *Resist the temptation.* It spells certain failure. If anything, overspend in the beginning since you can always cut back later. But if you underspend early, you'll never reach the *threshold of repetition* necessary to fly.

One Co-Op's Results—There are success stories around. Look at the case of 42 professionals who joined together to promote in the southern California media market. But it took expertise at the helm; 6- to 12-month contracts and notes; monthly prepayments; a small steering committee; $975 per month dues for a monthly budget of almost $41,000; sensible territories; a strong media mix; and excellent advertising. In the co-op's first 18 months, the program produced over 20,000 new patients, just under 50 new patients per month per practitioner.

☐ SPECIALISTS VS. GENERALISTS: THE BATTLE HEATS UP

The battle for business is growing, especially between specialists and generalists. For example, allergists now find that many other doctors do most of their own patients' allergy work.

These turf battles will almost surely grow. The generalist's strategy is clear—gain more expertise and promote that to existing patients and to the public at large. But for the specialist, the road is unclear.

Expanding Services—Specialists can combat the generalists by beating them at their own game. By expanding services, specialists can accept and keep more patients while still emphasizing their specialty. Undertaking this strategy requires delicacy to avoid shutting off the generalist's referral spigot. But in the long run, if done well, it assures volume.

Otherwise, specialists can become even more specialized, staying on the cutting edge of their work. If generalists keep the routine cases, specialists must stay *far enough ahead* of the pack to get all the difficult cases. In this case, a professional relations program to convince generalists of your level of expertise is mandatory.

The worst strategy is to do nothing. With the environment changing, if you do nothing, your practice slowly dwindles down. So act from strength. Not from desperation.

■ CHAPTER 11
Other Innovative Ways To Profitably Reach New Patients Now

☐ SIGNS OF THE TIMES

Northwest physician T.M. felt he wasn't capitalizing on the 7,100 cars that passed his freestanding office every day. Although he had a 60 × 24-in. "Physician" sign across the building's top facing, rarely did new patients indicate the sign as the reason for considering his practice. What to do?

Professionals often ask where they can get the best return on a marketing dollar invested. And most are surprised to learn it's their outdoor sign. For a one-time investment, your outside office sign can continually capture drive-by and walk-by traffic. If it's well done, no other media can do so much for so long for so little. In this case, with such a high volume of people passing by, T.M. has a ready-for-harvest opportunity.

Exposure—Outside signs need to be positioned for the greatest viewing exposure. To find the optimal sign location, stand in front of your office, and walk 50 ft in one direction. Stop and think where you'd put the sign to gain the greatest visibility. Is it curbside at eye level? Or on a 12-ft pole? Or set back? Or angled out from the facing? Snap photos from each stop to show your sign designers.

Go another 100 ft and repeat the process. Then another 100 ft. Now cross the street, and study your sign needs from there. Then walk back on that side of the street, and repeat the process at 100, 200, 300, 400, and 500 ft. Then cross back to the same side of the street as your office is on, and study the setting from there. Now walk back past your office, and stop every hundred feet on both sides of the street in that direction, taking pictures at each place.

131

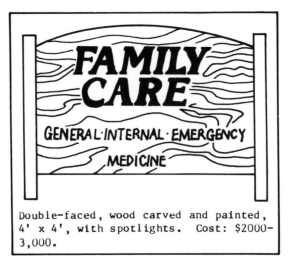

Double-faced, wood carved and painted, 4' x 4', with spotlights. Cost: $2000–3,000.

FIG 11–1.

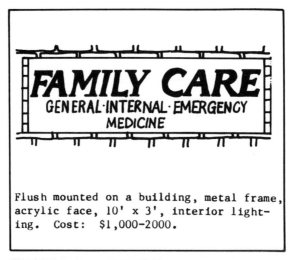

Flush mounted on a building, metal frame, acrylic face, 10' x 3', interior lighting. Cost: $1,000–2000.

FIG 11–2.

This short exercise will quickly make it clear where your sign should be placed for maximum exposure. Remember to check city and landlord regulations to be in compliance.

Design—Signs must pop out of the background. That doesn't mean Las Vegas neon, but it does mean breaking the visual plane. Look at Figures 11–1 through 11–9 to see the variation possible. The real trick is to establish the right image for the practice while grabbing attention. You and your sign designer have seven elements with which to work:

- *Height and location*: Ground level or raised. On the building or off. Curbside or recessed. Angled or flush.
- *Size*: Usually the bigger the sign, the more notice it gains. But size doesn't mean garishness, just effectiveness. The artwork determines the image, the size doesn't.
- *Color*: If you can, avoid using the same colors as everyone else to avoid becoming lost in the background.

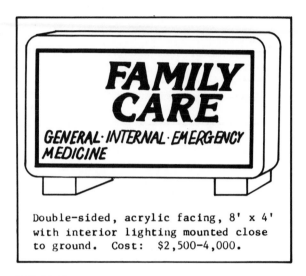

Double-sided, acrylic facing, 8' x 4' with interior lighting mounted close to ground. Cost: $2,500-4,000.

FIG 11-3.

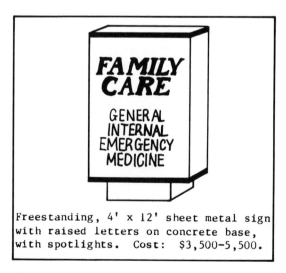

Freestanding, 4' x 12' sheet metal sign with raised letters on concrete base, with spotlights. Cost: $3,500-5,500.

FIG 11-4.

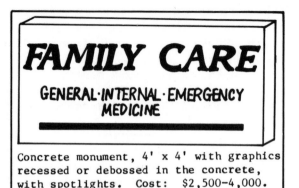

Concrete monument, 4' x 4' with graphics recessed or debossed in the concrete, with spotlights. Cost: $2,500-4,000.

FIG 11-5.

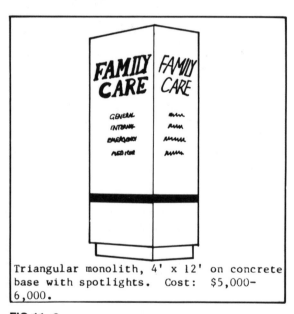

Triangular monolith, 4' x 12' on concrete base with spotlights. Cost: $5,000-6,000.

FIG 11-6.

- *Movement*: More expensive, but a real eye grabber. Turning on a pole. Electronic messages moving across a LED display. Even time and temperature.
- *Lighting*: Interior lighting or spotlights means the sign works 20 hours each day, not 12.
- *Shape*: Be unpredictable. An oval sign in a square sign environment. Freestanding monoliths when everyone else's is rectangular. Or molded in some distinctive shape.
- *Materials*: Wood, acrylic or other plastics, metal, concrete,

electric, painted, or some combination of those materials. Don't be a look-alike.

Copy—Breaking the visual plane gets your sign noticed. But what you say convinces them to come in. So even though the copy needs to be short, it needs to be convincing. Tell them what differentiates you from your competitors down the street. Experience, special expertise, affordability, hours, a full array of services, and so on. Your main distinction should go on the sign.

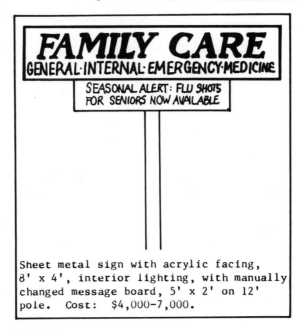

FIG 11–7.

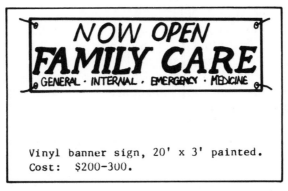

FIG 11–8.

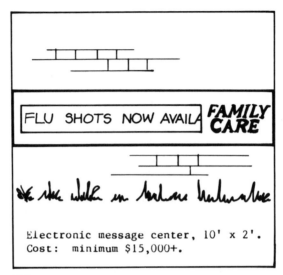

Electronic message center, 10' x 2'.
Cost: minimum $15,000+.

FIG 11–9.

For instance, in general medicine, the sign could read, "The Family Health Center for All Your Family's Needs." In psychiatry, "Short and Long Term Psychiatry—Over 20 years experience."

Construction—Any good local sign company can handle the manufacture and installation. But different companies certainly don't charge the same. The major trade magazine for the sign industry, *Signs of the Times*, recently bid a sign project out to 16 different shops. What did they find? The bids ranged from $1,170 to $5,355 for exactly the same job. The smart strategy: Shop heavily.

Results—After walking his sidewalks to determine location and viewing angles, it was simple for T.M. to envision a freestanding sign near the sidewalk in front of his recessed building. The size needed to be large, not only for attention but also for a feeling of being solid and competent. The result was a monolithic sign 4 ft wide by 12 ft high, made of wood, carved and painted, with spotlights for nighttime. The copy read "Total Family Health Care" to position the practice, with an illustration of a silhouetted family and T.M.'s name and credentials at the bottom.

Several days after the sign was installed, a new patient filling out the intake sheet answered "sign" to the question, "How did you learn of the practice?" The first month's tally was six new patients with a follow-up analysis showing gross receipts of $1,625 from those six. T.M.'s office went unnoticed by passing prospective patients no longer.

☐ EXPANSION BY BUYING ANOTHER PRACTICE

In corporate America, it's not uncommon for one company to gobble up a hard-pressed competitor to gain its assets or market share—and in the process to pay less than the going rate. With the rising cost of acquiring new patients, practitioners are increasingly turning to this same strategy. Expansion by purchase works exceedingly well in a number of situations. You can use it to buy more patients to gain market share. If you do, you *must* use a transition strategy to convert 70% or more of the practice's cases into your active file.

When you look at a practice that's for sale, consider the age of the charts, what percentage of them are active, and whether contact has been maintained over the years through mailings, calls, recalls, and so on. The older the charts and the less the communication, the less their value.

Sometimes you can buy the charts without the office. Prices for records alone vary between $1 and $25 each, depending on age, degree of commitment to the practice, and how well you bargain. If a practitioner is reduced to selling records as opposed to the entire practice, you can bargain hard on the price.

Purchasing the competition also stops another competitor from coming into that practice. These days, new professionals know that to launch, they must spend. So they line up their resources and promotional plan ahead of time. That means a big gun could buy the practice if you don't because the competition knows that promoting to an existing practice is less difficult and expensive than a cold start-

---

☐ Get A Free Ride

Insert your promotional material in every bill or mailing you send out. Use descriptions of new services, reminders about old ones, as well as manufacturers' brochures.

The "buck slip" format is inexpensive and works well. About the size of a dollar bill (hence, its name), it has room for information and a photo or illustration. Print both sides if you need.

As long as the insert doesn't increase the postage of the mailing, you're getting it sent for free. If the mailing in which you're enclosing the insert had to be sent anyway, your practice is ahead.

Also consider this. Place a message *on* every bill, statement, or recall you send. Put a message about the importance of recalls or checkups, an educational message, extended hours, new payment options, and so on. Again, it's all free and builds repetition. And that builds retention.

---

up. So that threat disappears or is lessened when you become the new owner. Nice, very nice.

Here's a third reason to buy a practice to expand. How do you grow when there are too many competitors in your area? Certainly there are ways, but these are more costly with a lower return on investment. Another approach is to go to a less competitive market. You could buy a practice in an area with a lower physician to population ratio and move there lock, stock, and barrel. Or you could purchase a practice there and have it as a second location.

Buying Tip— When you buy, consider a participatory buy-out. This means that a small initial payment is made for the practice with the larger dollars coming later. And those dollars should be dependent on how well the practice does. The better the gross, the more the seller receives.

This protects you in two ways. First, it keeps cash-in-hand when you need it most—at the start. There's nothing worse for a new practice, like any small business, than to be undercapitalized in the beginning.

Second, it saves you from being fooled. You never really know what you're buying until you've bought it. Only then do you fully understand the problems and opportunities. If you've really bought a "dog," with a participatory buy-out, your loss won't be crushing.

☐ HOW TO RETAIN PATIENTS WHEN YOU BUY A PRACTICE

D.L. was understandably ecstatic when he bought his first practice. He was buying from a retiring doctor who had practiced for 38 years, had well over 10,000 charts—rooms of them—and was the best-known and respected practitioner in the county.

The week of the transition, D.L. sent out a card announcing he had taken over the practice and new patients were being accepted. He also placed a professional announcement in the local daily and weekly newspapers. And he changed the name of the office to his own. All of these tactics made perfect sense to him and were consistent with the advice given by both a colleague and his office manager.

The exodus began at once. When the patients found out the former practitioner was gone, a full 16% who were calling for appointments decided to go elsewhere, with most going to a new heavily advertised clinic just down the street. As the weeks progressed and more people found out the doctor they had trusted so much was no logner available, fewer and fewer stayed with the practice. They felt their reason for coming was no longer there.

By Contrast—A.K. found himself in virtually the same situation, but by handling it differently, he actually saw patient flow rise by the third week after he took over. What had he done?

A.K. created a game plan to market himself to the former practitioner's patients. He was smart enough to realize their allegiance was to his predecessor—a loyalty he needed to transfer *in toto* to himself. Here were the steps in his game plan.

Letter 1: As part of the negotiated deal, the former practitioner had agreed to sign a letter A.K. would write. Mailed to all his patients, this two-page letter announced he was retiring. He wrote that treating his patients had fulfilled him more than he could tell them. And that he wanted to thank each one of them for giving him that opportunity.

He then wrote about how a lengthy search had been made to find a new practitioner to care for his patients. The search had not been easy because he had always felt that their health care was a sacred responsibility. He could not entrust their records to just any qualified physician—only a very special one. Even though many physicians were available, the right one with the right schooling, training, credentials, experience, and manner proved difficult to find.

But now the search was over. The former practitioner then lauded A.K.'s background and reiterated how much he could be trusted. A photo of the two physicians shaking hands and smiling appeared at the top of the letter.

Letter 2: A week later, A.K. sent his own two-page follow-up letter. It praised the former practitioner and explained how difficult it will be to fill his shoes. He then stated how fortunate he felt to have been selected by the retiring doctor and entrusted with the patient's records and health. To him, he explained, this is a professional trust. And the patient could feel assured that he or she would continue to receive the kind of service and treatment given in the past.

A.K. then described the improved, new state-of-the-art treatment he would provide because of recent breakthroughs he had mastered and the new services he'd made available—including new convenient extended office hours. This letter, too, had a photo, but a different one, of the two physicians smiling and shaking hands. The photos helped transfer the good feelings about the former practitioner to his successor. A.K. also included telephone stickers for the patient's phone, rolodex, and personal address books.

The Practice Name Transition—A.K. also changed the practice name as D.L. had, but A.K. kept the former practitioner's name associated with the practice. In fact, he simply added his name on the end for

Rethinking Holiday Cards

"Ho, ho, ho" is the gleeful response of holiday card companies as they sell tons of their holiday cards to professionals who will send them to patients with the intent of spreading goodwill while promoting their practices.

But analyze for a moment what these well-meaning greetings really achieve. The average person receives enough holiday cards to wallpaper the living room. But if the person were asked to recite who had sent all the cards, chances are only a few friends and family names would be remembered. Your sizable expenditure is better dispensed elsewhere.

But even though your holiday cards don't affect most people, they do have an impact on some. You can identify who those patients are by noticing which ones send you cards. Keep mailing cards to them. If you don't know who they are, compile your list from this year's cards, and reciprocate for each card you get.

A Better Strategy.—If you want your goodwill remembered, look for opportunities where competition for attention is far less intense, such as a birthday.

But if you feel you *must* send holiday cards, do mail early. The week *before* Thanksgiving is best since the rest of the wallpaper hasn't hit the mails yet. And take the money out of your charity budget, not promotion.

---

the first 12 months. Then he switched his to the front for the next 12 months before dropping the older practitioner's name altogether. This further transferred, by association, all those years of positivity to A.K.

Results—The strategy worked beautifully. The kudos of the former practitioner enhanced the new physician's image. The emphasis on trust, cooperation, being handpicked, plus the added services that emphasized the new and improved struck a meaningful chord in patients.

Repetition of the message also worked. First one letter, then another. And then every 3 months, A.K. religiously sent a two-page letter talking about new developments for his patients to know about and to take advantage of. These letters drove home the message that A.K. was progressive and caring.

The bottom line? Dollar volume went up 27% in the first 3 months instead of the usual beginning doldrums. And now since the patient base was being communicated with, patients who had not returned in five years did so now.

"It was just a matter of putting myself in these patients' shoes and figuring out why they stayed with that practitioner. Once I did that, I capitalized on that trust and thought of ways to transfer it over."

☐ CONVERTING BUSINESS CARDS INTO PROMOTION

What's the purpose of your business card? Most practitioners would answer that it's an easy way to give someone your address and phone number. Others who rarely give them out can't come up with a good reason—just that you're supposed to have them.

Both answers treat them as an expense and both ignore the opportunities they represent. But in practice, your business card can be an additional way to convince people to come to you.

Business cards haven't traditionally been seen as potent promoters. Name, address, and phone number alone fall far short of encouraging anyone to act. So to turn your cards from an expense into an income generator, treat it like an ad. Use sharp graphics, and use the card to tell prospective patients why they should come to you.

Short Copy—Limit your promotional copy to one or two lines or phrases that state or imply the strong benefit you offer. No more. Writing short, potent copy where every word counts is not always easy. In fact, in copywriting, there's an old adage, "If I'd had the time, I'd have written it shorter." Good advice: Take the time.

Some successful one-liners:

- Experience you can trust.
- Exclusively serving men and women in high-stress positions within the executive, management, and professional community.
- Childbirth to suit your wishes. Hospital. Home. Alternative birth centers.
- Emphasizing short-term therapy for individuals and families.
- We care about your child.
- You'll take pride in our results—and your new appearance (plastic surgeons).

Combine Copy With Graphics—Choose a graphic treatment that does three things: (1) It should get the card noticed and read; (2) it should convey the proper image for your practice; (3) it should expand on the copy and validates it or convey additional benefits. Well-done logos, pictures, drawings, or simply a clean layout with some artistic enhancements can be used.

Strive for an understated elegance that conveys quality. To achieve this, emphasize what art directors call "white space," an uncluttered look that avoids having the card crammed with type. Add a clean, easy-to-read, professional-looking typeface. Then print in elegant color combinations: light gray paper with maroon or navy ink; white stock with dark green or blue and gold ink; ivory stock with navy, dark green, or dark brown ink. The paper should be coated or have a linen or laid texture, which also conveys a quality image. Also acceptable but not a "stopper": a flat vellum finish.

Passing Them Out— Some professionals go so far as to create the perfect promotional card but then let them go to waste by not distributing them. Obviously, the cards can't promote your practice unless you distribute them. How to hand them out? Simple. Everyone you meet, ask for their card. And they'll ask for yours in return. The wider the distribution, the bigger the return.

☐ WELCOME WAGON: BOOM OR BUST?

Want to attract new residents, new parents, or the newly engaged to your practice and have your message presented personally to these prospective patients in a tasteful and dignified manner? Without the less sensitive, impersonal approach of advertising in newspapers, *Yellow Pages*, or other media? And, above all, discreetly?

These are the claims of the Welcome Wagon, the more than 50-year-old organization famous for greeting new residents and representing local retail establishments. Sensing an opportunity, the Wel-

---

☐ Business Card Analysis: Positioning As A Specialist

Louis Alpern is more than an ophthalmologist. He's a specialist in cataracts and glaucoma. It's true that practically all general ophthalmologists treat these two conditions, but by positioning himself as a specialist, he'll garner more of that business.

On his business card, shown in Figure 11–10, the name of his practice can act as the headline because it contains the promise of specialization and greater ability. The strong modern graphics reinforce his specialization and get the card read. Notice how the graphics take up 40% of the card. With the addition of a few credentials, the card successfully represents the ability of the practitioner.

Dr. Alpern also knows whom he treats. On the flip side, seen in Figure 11–11, is a translation for his Spanish-speaking patients. This is a far better execution to reach Spanish-speaking prospective patients than simply putting both on the same side or adding "se habla espanol." To Anglos, it means he specializes in them. To Latinos, it means the same.

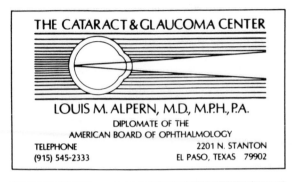

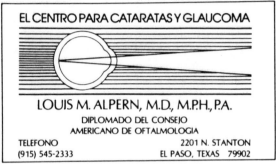

FIGS 11–10 (top) and 11–11 (bottom).

come Wagon has now designed a program expressly for the medical, dental, legal, and veterinary fields. But does the Welcome Wagon's formula repackaged for the professional really work?

The Practice Builder interviewed 25 practitioners across the country to find out about the program and its effectiveness. Here's what was discovered:

1. New move-ins and prospects undergoing life-style changes do often need a new cadre of professionals. The Welcome Wagon targets those lucrative segments—a positive factor.

2. The Welcome Wagon reps make a presentation on behalf of the practice, help design the sales message to be presented, the advertising specialty to be left behind as a reminder, and the invitation to visit the practice. However, most reps' knowledge of professional marketing and their planning ability was minimal at best. So the strategies and execution were far from optimal—a negative factor.

3. The Welcome Wagon program was publicized locally to stimulate results—a plus factor.

4. The representatives had difficulty attracting professionals into the program so there was little competition in the Welcome Wagon basket—another plus factor.

5. The professional received the names, addresses, and phone numbers of those visited. Results depend on effective follow-up by the professional—a positive factor.

6. The reps can't solicit business on behalf of the professional. Instead, the professional is a sponsor of the program. This all-important difference between "discreet sponsorship" and bottom-line results depends on the rep. The program guidelines say they don't solicit. But at $2 per call times 20 calls per month, the program costs $480 a year. At that price, the pitch may be discreet, but the results must be concrete.

Bottom Line—Of the 25 professionals surveyed, 9 reported respectable or promising results. Sixteen said, "Never again." The Welcome Wagon program played better in the East than in the West. Perhaps as one rep said, "The West Coast isn't community-oriented enough."

What differentiated the winners from the losers? Two variables. First, the abilities of the rep. If the rep knows how to sell (while keeping one eye on the "no soliciting" guideline) and has a high

---

☐ Promotions In Motion

To spur your own creativity, here are some successful special promotions being used today. When reading the examples, first consider your market's need in addition to your own needs. Not all ideas are transferable, but the list should plant and nurture some promotional seeds:

■ A Florida ophthalmologist has nondriving patients chauffeured by van to the office.

■ In New Jersey, a practitioner runs on-screen ads at local movie theatres to promote his practice. Analysis: unorthodox and a bit expensive to produce the commercial, but highly effective.

■ A podiatric partnership in Florida provides coffee and wine in the waiting room to provide a relaxed atmosphere for anxious patients. And every patient who has had any kind of procedure is also called that evening by one of the doctors.

■ A general practitioner in Maryland offers free checkups for those just engaged or newly married. He's not only seen an increase in his practice from his direct mail program promoting the checkups (the mailing list is from newspaper announcements and marriage license issuances), but after 3 years, many of these initial checkups have turned into obstetric cases. The targeting of this group has produced long-term patients as well as raising his recognition and stature in the community. And that's increased the response to his *Yellow Pages* ad and other promotions.

energy level, that's half the battle. The other key is follow-up. Phoning, mailing, mailing, and phoning again all work. Welcome Wagon opens the door; repetition brings them in.

Check First—Before signing up, check the results other professionals have had—not with the Welcome Wagon in general, but with your rep in particular.

■ PART 2   Your Tools

■ SECTION 3
Turning To Advertising: Spending Your Money Instead Of Your Time To Attract New Patients

■ CHAPTER 12
Should You Advertise? If So, Where?

☐ DOES ADVERTISING HURT YOUR IMAGE?

Does advertising mean you need business? And if it does mean you need business, is that a sign that you're an inferior practitioner? This is a concern that's privately voiced everyday by doctors—but *only* by nonadvertising practitioners.

Recent studies show that when asked about professionals who advertise, the public's approval rate is over 70%. That's a bigger landslide than Reagan's.

Professionals who advertise don't worry about this issue. They count their receipts or lick their wounds, depending on their ability to promote.

Creating an Image—Does advertising hurt your image? Does it hurt Mercedes-Benz' image? Or Cartier's? Hardly. In fact, it *creates* the image.

The only time that advertising could hurt your image is from poor execution. Beware of looking like "dollar days" at K-Mart.

☐ WHAT'S YOUR TRUE BOTTOM LINE

Dr. D.F. hired an ad agency to create two direct mail packages— one targeting local residents, the other to generate patient flow from among employees of local businesses. Problem: When D.F. read the agency's first drafts, he felt the copy was too aggressive for his taste— even though the image was dignified.

Doze and Don't— D.F. called the agency to complain. And he drafted his own sample letters to show the agency the tone and posture he wanted. Agency's problem: D.F.'s version was so low-key and un-motivating, it could have easily won FDA approval as a tranquilizer.

The agency explained that profitable direct mail must convey a sense of excitement and urgency about it, that the vocabulary was carefully chosen to reinforce that feeling and to appeal to the reader's emotions as well as the mind.

What's Really the Point?—D.F. hadn't thought through his real reason for the promotion. Ostensibly, it was to produce patient flow and profits. But if that had been his true bottom line, D.F. would let the agency create the projects based on proven concepts and techniques.

Instead, his watered-down versions hinted at two other unconscious goals. First, he wanted to satisfy a nagging feeling that he should do something about building his practice. Like so many other professionals, D.F. didn't quite know what it should be—as long as he didn't *lose* money. Second, D.F. was wary of a promotion that might ruffle the feathers of his colleagues.

Unfortunately, making profits and these two other bottom line goals are incompatible. Launching a lukewarm promotion just for the sake of doing something will usually guarantee its failure. On the other hand, if a promotion is successful, then colleagues—or more bluntly put, competitors—will feel ruffled. After all, they're threatened with a loss of business.

Decision—By identifying the real reason for creating a promotion, the tenor of its execution becomes clearer, no longer at cross purposes. And if you find your bottom line muddled, here's *The Practice Builder's* advice: Forget the promotion—it won't be effective. You might as well take the money and spend it on a Club Med vacation.

☐ TEN COMMON MISTAKES IN ADVERTISING

Why waste your advertising dollars? Here are some simple lessons that have taken big business billions of dollars to learn the hard way. Advertising pro Alec Benn came up with a list of *The 27 Most Common Mistakes in Advertising* [1] committed by large corporate advertisers. But several of the points have application to professionals advertising their practices. We've pointed out many of them elsewhere, but they bear repeating. Save your time and money by avoiding these common mistakes:

1. *"Putting a person in charge of your advertising whose job responsibilities do not coincide with the purpose of advertising"*: For example, don't appoint your office manager to oversee advertising; his or her major responsibilities are focused on ensuring that the office runs efficiently. They haven't anything to do with increasing patient flow. Instead, accurately define the purpose of the advertising you want to do, and this will help you select the proper person to oversee it. Since you have the greatest stake in your practice, we advise that you have final responsibility.

2. *"Choosing an advertising agency with the wrong expertise"*: Building a practice isn't the same thing as selling cookies or boosting magazine renewals. Instead, ask prospective agencies about their experience with other professionals and companies with services that are marketed in the same way as your own. Then take the time to educate the agency about yourself, your practice, and your patients.

3. *"Trying to do too much with too few advertising dollars"*: Instead, concentrate your advertising budget on the one or two most effective media for your services.

4. *"Choosing a medium for your advertising based on its low rate and total cost, rather than on the cost per thousand readers, listeners, or viewers"*: Instead, compare audience sizes as well as cost. In advertising, the common yardstick is the cost per thousand (CPM), that is, how much it costs an advertiser to reach a thousand readers, listeners, or viewers. To come up with the figure, divide the audience size (in thousands) into the total cost of the advertising vehicle. For example:

☐ Newspaper A:

$$\frac{\$581 \text{ cost of ad}}{51.8 \text{ (thousands)}} \; = \; \$11.21 \text{ CPM}$$

☐ Newspaper B:

$$\frac{\$720 \text{ cost of ad}}{72.9 \text{ (thousands)}} \; = \; \$9.87 \text{ CPM}$$

When seen in these terms, although Newspaper B does cost more, it's the better buy.

5. *"Not advertising frequently enough"*: Instead, run your ad long enough for it to have an effect. Remember that all media are saturated with advertisements and only a fraction of the audience will recall your ad the following day.

6. *"Making an advertisement bigger than it needs to be"*: Remember that reader attention is captured at a diminishing rate once an ad more

than dominates a page. Instead, small can be beautiful and effective. Test different sized ads—a fourth of a page and a half page—for response.

7. *"Expecting too much from creativity in copy and art"*: Instead, make your prospective patients an offer they can't refuse—it might be unusual value or the care and other important attributes they look for in a physician. And make the offer over and over again. Even famous ads such as Volkswagen's "Think Small" campaign would have failed had not the product been worthwhile and the ad itself repeated many times to ensure its memorability.

8. *"Imitating instead of analyzing"*: Instead, be sure your advertising is unique and tailored to your needs. Consider the following:

- The purpose of your ad
- The nature of your audience
- The demographics of your audience
- The media you're using
- The nature of your services
- Your competition
- *"Entertaining instead of selling"*: Advertising's reason for being is too sell, not amuse. The ad doesn't need to scream, but it does need to sell. The following adage in advertising tells what success is attributed to: "40% is because of *what* you say, 40% is because of *who* you say it to, and only 20% is due to *how* you say it."
- *"Failing to fully utilize the peculiar advantages of the medium"*: Examples are not being visual enough on television or not creating strong mental pictures on radio. Instead, use copywriters or creative directors who are skilled in the medium you are using.
- *"An advertiser handling direct mail yourself without retaining the necessary experts"*: Instead, use the experts. Direct mail is an

---

☐ What Should Your Advertising Pay?

The Practice Builder's rule: Every $10 spent on advertising should yield $100 in increased billings. Breaking even is not a successful campaign. Rather than break even, it would make more sense to put your ad budget in the bank so that you'd at least get the interest on the money. When you invest in advertising, improve your strategies, differentiate yourself from the competition, find a new audience or target market. Make it work so it can return the dividends it should.

---

effective, but difficult area of advertising, and trying to do it yourself could cost you a lot more than the money you think you might save.

- *"Believing advertising is more powerful than it really is"*: Realize that it takes a lot more to create a successful practice than successful ads. You need all those other elements—good care, pricing, location, and more—in place before you run a good ad.

☐ DIRECT RESPONSE VS. NAME RECOGNITION

Ohio family practitioner G.A. mailed 8,200 pieces of direct mail to households with a message that essentially said, "When you need a physician, remember my name." With only six responses and two new patients, G.A. never did another advertising campaign. Cost: $2,960. Immediate loss: $2,810.

A California orthopedic surgeon, however, did succeed—temporarily. He sent out 10,000 Val-Pac cooperative coupons offering a free foot exam. With 18 responses and 4 surgeries, he generated $2,800 in billings on a $300 investment. That 933% return in 90 days certainly seemed a sure-footed strategy.

But this became his sole promotional effort. As he repeatedly flooded his upper-middle income, white-collar market with coupons, many of his older, more affluent patients began slowly to see him as a low-end clinic. They stopped coming in.

Two Strategies—Both doctors made serious mistakes because they failed to understand the tactics required for long-term success with the promotional strategy they chose.

There are essentially two broad stroke strategies available—name recognition and direct response. In name recognition, the physician promotes the practice in some form of advertising or public relations effort that repeats the practice's name and frequently shows the logo. The purpose is recall. When prospective patients are looking for a new physician, they'll remember your name or recognize it in the *Yellow Pages*.

Remembering the Name—With name recognition, the advertising has no offers to spur response now. But there is a requirement for its success: that you do lots and lots of name-recognition advertising and promotion over the long term. This strategy succeeds only if the practice has a strong, unwavering commitment to the long haul.

Why? Because the response curve is slow in rising. Yet while it may start slowly, it will rise steadily. If the promotion stops down the road, the responses keep on coming in, needing only minimal additional efforts to maintain the curve.

So with name recognition, the practitioner must persevere. With little immediate response in the beginning and money continually being invested, most practitioners who don't understand the dynamics get nervous and pull the promotional plug before the curve has enough time to swing up.

So understanding, money, and fortitude are the name of the game. But often the budget—and your stomach lining—can't handle the wait. For those who can, however, name recognition builds the solid, long-term practice with an impeccable image.

Name Recognition Tactics— G.A., the Ohio family practitioner, chose this strategy, but unfortunately, he also chose the wrong tactic in executing the strategy. Frequent repetition can be accomplished with direct mail, but because of the initial cost, it's not often the vehicle of choice.

Instead, prolific public relations efforts or small but continuous space advertising in newspapers or magazines or on radio or TV is preferable. Buy small space so the budget can handle it and continuous spots so you're there when they need you.

Direct Response—Today, many practitioners use a direct response strategy because the budget requirements are less and the responses come in immediately. At the very heart of direct response is an offer— something free, dollars off, loss leaders, additional services at discounted prices, gifts or premiums. These are the same tactics retail businesses have traditionally turned to when they need foot traffic *now*. And they work, whether in direct mail, newspapers, shoppers, magazines, or on radio or television.

With direct response, you avoid the need for the big expenditures of a name recognition campaign while getting acceptable and immediate returns. This type of promotion can give your practice a quick boost during a slump, but it normally doesn't produce a pool of highly loyal patients. Also, as in the case with the California orthopedic surgeon, there is a downside risk: your image.

The risk is hard to perceive because image is so difficult to measure. And direct response is seductive because of the immediate cash flow. Fortunately, there is a way to balance the program and avoid becoming seen as a price-cutter.

First, use your offer as a closing tool. This means you lead your promotions with other strong, nonprice benefits that your price provides. Thus the coupon or offer becomes a low-risk way of obtaining these other benefits.

☐ Ad Analysis: Strong Image Builder

How do you say "I care" in an ad? Lots of ads simply say, "I care . . . I care . . . I care," but they don't communicate the essence of caring when they used that hackneyed phrase without backing it up.

But the ad in Figure 12–1 is different. First the professionally taken photograph of the doctor captures the readers' attention and sets the tone of concern. Then the headline quote compresses the message into four words— nice tight writing.

The remainder of the copy gives support to the claim by explaining Dr. Harris's philosophy that says it all and says it without once using the phrase, "I care."

Also look at that second paragraph and how it presents his discounts for certain patients. Rather than damaging his image by portraying the practice as a low-end clinic, the discounts build his image and reinforce the caring message.

Slight Improvement.—There's a need to target the population better— those people who need an otolaryngologist. If you wait until the second paragraph, you'll lose many prime readers because only 25% will read the body copy. Therefore, we usually recommend targeting in the headline or visual. In this case, the best place is in the photo caption that would read:

Norman J. Harris, M.D.
Ear, Nose & Throat Specialist
Orange, California

Remember, image-building ads such as this one need to be run continuously throughout the next 6 to 12 months before you'll get a strong response. Then, most likely, it will show up as an increased response to the *Yellow Pages*. So make sure your *Yellow Pages* presence is solid.

Good photo, good ad, good luck.

This avoids price being the only point of differentiation from your competitors. And it gives the public other benefits from which to form their image of you. And the offer of a discounted initial visit—or whatever the offer is—can be made to a well-defined group of prospective patients in the interest of their health and well-being. For example, in late summer, a pediatrician could offer reduced fees on the inoculations needed to enroll a child in kindergarten. Such a discount can actually benefit the physician's image when the offer is shown as a public service gesture to ensure that the children receive the vaccinations they need.

Second, engage in nonprice promotions, either through public relations or name-recognition advertising. These strengthen your community image the same way. Between the two tactics, image damage should not be a problem.

Your Choice— Which strategy is best for you? That depends on your budget, nerves, and personal likes. But whichever you choose, be consistent.

☐ SHOULD YOU PRICE ADVERTISE?

Price advertising doesn't make sense in most competitive situations, but it does in some. Medicine, of course, has historically been immune to the fate of supermarkets where it's become very difficult to avoid price advertising because all the competition is doing it. Then

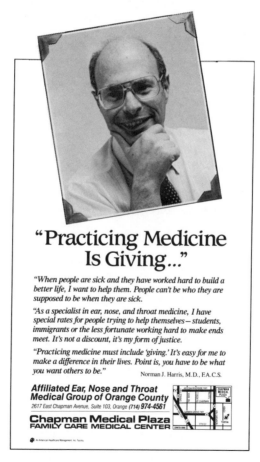

"Practicing Medicine Is Giving..."

"When people are sick and they have worked hard to build a better life, I want to help them. People can't be who they are supposed to be when they are sick.

"As a specialist in ear, nose, and throat medicine, I have special rates for people trying to help themselves—students, immigrants or the less fortunate working hard to make ends meet. It's not a discount, it's my form of justice.

"Practicing medicine must include 'giving.' It's easy for me to make a difference in their lives. Point is, you have to be what you want others to be." Norman J. Harris, M.D., F.A.C.S.

Affiliated Ear, Nose and Throat Medical Group of Orange County
2617 East Chapman Avenue, Suite 103, Orange **(714) 974-4561**

Chapman Medical Plaza
FAMILY CARE MEDICAL CENTER

FIG 12–1.

the public begins to suspect all the claims of low cost, and almost all the markets need to price advertise.

Many professions today have practitioners whose advertisements look much like a supermarket ad with their screaming claims of low cost. In a couple of instances, this is appropriate. Some lawyers, veterinarians, dentists, optometrists, and others have taken to price advertising when they found themselves in very competitive markets and realized that the competition wasn't filling the needs of the cost-conscious. Usually the first practitioner to price advertise in a market discovers two things. One is that he or she will largely be successful. And two, that the competitors will dislike your actions since they correctly see the threat to their own business. One must decide whether the potential profits made are really worth the slings and arrows.

One other situation prime for price advertising is when you've nothing to lose. If the practice is in a death dive, pull out all the stoppers. You're not concerned about image at this point, nor the long term. Just an immediate influx of cash. And aggressive price advertising will do just that.

Cautions—Price advertising is designed to cast out a net and haul in a load of fish so you can pick out the few big ones. But there are quite a large number of small fish too. Prepare the staff for the influx. Price sensitive patients will flood your waiting room.

Streamline your handling of these patients to find the big cases to which you can then devote your time. Schedule their initial visits at less desirable times, or lump them together so the whole office goes into high gear for serving the numbers. Problem: If the staff isn't ready *and agreeable*, their passive-aggressive behavior will sabotage your effort.

How to Price Advertise—How you price advertise determines whom you attract and the practice's profit margin. A "free" anything brings in the most responses—but the least qualified patients. Many can't afford you. So their loyalty is less and the volume may frazzle you and the staff. But the number of large cases may be big.

To attract patients who are more likely to be able to afford your services, test a reduced fee for a common service. The responses certainly aren't as high as offering a free something, but those who do come are better patients.

Rarely do you find a total discount office in any profession. Those that do price advertise choose a popular service or product and offer it as a loss leader. They cut its price and take a loss on those they sell in the hopes that the patient or client will buy other services at their standard fee.

There is room in the marketplace for a total discount medical office. Those who choose this route have two important factors. They must allocate sufficient resources for constant promotion. And second, costs must be kept to the bone. Without a watchful eye on costs, thin margins erode quickly.

Price advertising is usually an option only for those unconcerned with their image or those who can't afford that nicety. On the other hand, one could argue that truly discounted services, promoted to those who would need them, would serve the public good. Providing well-priced medical services would help those, for example, who have inadequate insurance coverage and can't afford other physicians and yet aren't so poor that they qualify for public assistance.

REFERENCES

1. Benn A: *The 27 Most Common Mistakes in Advertising.* New York, AMA-COM, 1978, pp 138–142.

■ CHAPTER 13
Creating Your Quintessential Marketing Piece

☐ GETTING NOTICED IN THE CLUTTER

Each day the average adult hears or sees 2,000 commercial messages. They range from signs to television commercials to newspaper ads to direct mail and so on. And they're not just from Fortune 500 companies with household names but also from colleagues in your specialty. With that kind of information pollution, the mind simply can't process it all. Much of it is totally ignored. It isn't heard or seen.

Whether you're creating a public relations effort or an ad message, getting noticed seems impossible. How can you get your message across?

Create Your Own Dandelion—Look at the dandelions in your lawn. No matter how high the grass is, the dandelions always seem to pop higher. In short or long grass, the dandelions always stand out on top.

That's the challenge for small practitioners, advises Gunther Klaus, Ph.D.[1] Create a message that pops up from this information clutter. "It doesn't take dollars. It takes ingenuity. Make your messages strong and irresistible, and you'll be able to create your own dandelion. That's how you compete for attention against the big guys."

☐ THE DIFFERENCE BETWEEN HYPE AND SUBSTANCE

Having emphasized the importance of being noticed, let's temper it with a cry for substance. There is a belief that all you need to do in promotion is grab attention. It's interpreted to mean loud splashes

☐ **Six Key Words That Aid Your Writing²**

Before the first draft

1. Think
2. Plan
3. Organize

After the first draft

4. Revise
5. Revise
6. Revise

---

of noisy promotion that certainly attract attention, but also creates an *inappropriate image* for the professional.

We've all seen it in the newspapers—the retail-look ads that scream "$25 off exams." Or radio spots with two housewives having a conversation about a professional that leaves you with the impression that these are silly people with silly concerns. Or *Yellow Pages* ads that should inspire, but instead they're so distasteful, you want to expire.

Substance is Preferable—In the promotion of medical services, credibility is more important than any other attribute. Since everyone wants a "good" physician, building that credibility is mandatory to establish the right image in any advertising whether it's the *Yellow Pages*, shoppers, or even signs on the back of buses.

Ads that hype only may gain the attention they so desperately seek, but then they leave the prospective patient asking, "Well, now that you've got my attention, what do you have to say?" Credibility answers that question; hype doesn't.

Substance also comes in another form. Most professionals who do their own promotion simply duplicate what others have done previously. This happens so often that everyone begins to look alike. And the response to all the advertising dies.

You must differentiate yourself and show that you're credible —after you've gained their attention.

☐ CRITERIA FOR WINNING ADS

Wally Wood, editor of *Magazine Age,* recently served as a judge in the international professional communications awards competition sponsored by the Business/Professional Advertising Association. This is the big league. The 300 ads judged were among the best in the world.

Four Criteria—The following criteria are used in the big league. How do your ads compare?

1. *Visual impact—stopping power*: Does the headline and illustration compel reading?
2. *Identity*: Is it immediately apparent what's being advertised? You'd be surprised how often it isn't, even after close reading.
3. *Selling proposition*: Are good reasons for buying logically presented in terms of the benefits to prospects? Wood was surprised at the number of ads that gave no benefits whatsoever and forgot about logic. And these were among the potential prize winners.
4. *Effectiveness of overall creative effort vs. stated objective*: The ad's objectives should be clear and written before the creative effort is tackled.

Headline and Illustration Are Key—These two elements were judged most heavily since they are the most important elements in real-world competition. "Beware of the bad headline," warns Wood. Headlines in tricky type are impossible to read. Avoid headlines that are clever but say nothing. And avoid headlines that aren't clever and say nothing.

Test your ad against these criteria.

☐ AD ANALYSIS: SIMPLE AND DIRECT

The ad shown in Figure 13–1 demonstrates the importance of an ad's headline and its illustration. Designed for use in the *Yellow Pages,* the ad targets those very specific readers who are already looking in the directory for a dermatologist. So the headline zeros in on those with skin, scalp, or nail problems. The subhead then implies the benefit of seeing someone with the expertise needed. The subhead also flatters the reader by implying that the reader is special and deserves the attention of a specialist—"It is important for *you* to see a *specialist.*"

That and the friendly, smiling faces of the doctor and an attractive, mature patient reassure the reader that this specialist will be able to solve all the reader's problems. The remainder of the ad reinforces those images by including the procedures offered and then an impressive list of credentials.

Simple. Direct. Effective.

☐ EE = EO

EE = EO is a simple equation that means when you emphasize everything (EE), you emphasize nothing (EO). And the result is zero.

Too many ads drone because all the information is given the same weight. Think of a display ad with all the same-sized type, the radio spot that has the same emphasis throughout, the letter that lists every imaginable selling point but doesn't expound on any of them. In each of these cases, the message is there, but it's watered down and has no impact.

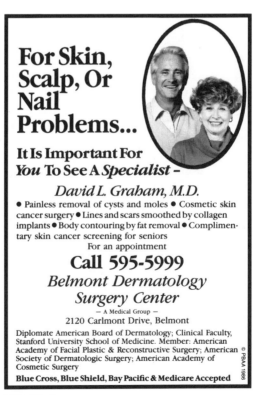

FIG 13–1.

☐ Keep It Simple

One advertiser[3] found that 43% of consumers didn't understand the word "obsolete." A brewer found that many customers thought "lagered" meant tired. And Procter & Gamble had to drop the word "concentrated" from its ads because many readers thought it meant "blessed by the Pope."
Strategy: Keep the language simple. Don't use technical or difficult words.

Ad tip: Emphasize one or two points in the headline. Have the copy expound on them and explain them. The more you tell about those one or two points, the more convincing it will be. Cover additional features in the copy, but don't give them the same emphasis. Those other points should be secondary.

☐ HOW TO WRITE BODY COPY

The average readership of the body of an ad is only about 5%. So the copy needs to be well written, or you'll lose that 1 in 20 who apparently was interested enough in what you had to say to read that far. Ad guru David Ogilvy suggests the following:

1. Don't address readers as though they were together in a stadium. When people read your copy, they're alone. Imagine that you're writing each of them a letter—one human being to another, second person singular.

2. You can't bore people into buying your service. You can only interest them into buying it. So think about them, not yourself.

3. It pays to avoid difficult words. When copywriters argue with Ogilvy about some arcane word they want to use, he tells them, "Get on a bus. Go to Iowa. Stay on a farm for a week, and and talk to the farmer. Come back to New York by train, and talk to your fellow passengers in the day coach. If you still want to use the word, go ahead."

4. Long copy outputs short copy. If it's interesting, even long copy, as long as 5,000 words, works better. Why? Because long copy may convey the impression that you have something important to say. And because the more facts you tell, the more you sell. But remember—if you write long copy, your first paragraph and the headline had better be grabbers.

☐ DOES YOUR AD HAVE A CREDIBILITY GAP?

Most practitioner's ads sound one of two ways—either dull and boring or so filled with superlatives as to be unbelievable. A remedy for both ailments is to quantify how you're the best, or whatever the claim, with the use of a statistic. Numbers have an authoritative ring to them that shows the reader you've tested your claim and can offer concrete evidence of it's validity.

Back Up Claims—That brings up another point about one critical need of any promotion. If your ad shows an advantage or makes a large claim, be sure that you back up that claim in the ad. Credibility is very important in any ad. When you state an advantage or benefit, also be sure to explain how you can deliver it. You can do it with statistics or offer other proof, but you've got to overcome the reader's skepticism before they'll trust you.

By the same token, any state disclaimer requirements should be handled carefully. Today, many sophisticated ads talk of successful case histories, implying that the reader can enjoy this same success. Some states require a disclaimer that the practitioner can't guarantee results.

No Small Type—It's best *not* to use asterisks and small type disclaimers at the bottom of the ad. The public will perceive them as there because of the legal requirement to protect readers against misleading statements. Instead, avoid that red flag and turn a negative into a positive—right in the copy. For example, say, "We don't accept all patients, but those we do accept almost always have excellent results. So to find out whether we can help you, please call us for a consultation. We'll be glad to discuss your situation and let you know whether we can count you among our success stories."

Needing to prove what you say even extends to the claim that

☐ Involving The Reader

Ads that involve the reader are effective. For example, an ad for a menopause clinic could read, "Menopause Affects Every Woman." But a better headline would be "A Critical Test If You're a Woman 45–55." The ad then has a checklist of menopausal symptoms and introduces the clinic. Another involvement headline: "What's wrong with this picture?" for substance abuse.

"we care." It's hard to find a professional brochure or ad that doesn't claim "we care." Unfortunately, it's also hard to find one that proves it, which means it's not believed and it's quickly dismissed. If you choose this "high touch" way to position your practice, satisfy all the people from Missouri who say, "Show me."

In the ad's graphics it means photos of the practitioner looking eye-to-eye and touching or being close to the patient. In the copy, it means telling the prospective patients that you take the time in this hurried world to understand each of them as an individual and treat them as important. That if you're backlogged, you call to tell them you're running 20 minutes late so there's no need for them to rush. That they are recognized when they come into the office because there aren't new assistants every time they come in. That you'll follow up after seeing them just to make sure everything's going according to plan. That when you make a referral, you'll call to make sure that they're happy with it.

Showing you care means you deliver on those promises—that you're available with convenient hours; that you write down your private or home number on your business card and give it out in appropriate situations; that you don't act rushed so that patients feel cheated.

If you really care, prove it—in your promotion and in your practice. Otherwise, talk about your equipment.

☐ AD ANALYSIS: ADDRESSING WORKADAY CONCERNS

Headlines that address bread-and-butter issues are almost always effective, particularly when they also promise solutions to the reader's concerns. And few concerns come closer to home than the question of how to be a better breadwinner.

The newspaper ad shown in Figure 13–2 is a good example of one that focuses on the almost universal concern of how to improve one's job performance. The subject is reinforced with photos showing two serious individuals hard at work—two serious individuals unhampered by glasses.

The copy expands and proves the headline by first discussing all of the disadvantages of glasses and contacts and then describing the new alternative. The use of the free seminar format is also a wise choice when discussing a subject that few readers are conversant with. But the prospective patient is nonetheless given a choice. Those who don't or can't attend the seminar can still receive a "fact-packed report" on RK.

This copy-protected ad should rate a high job performance.

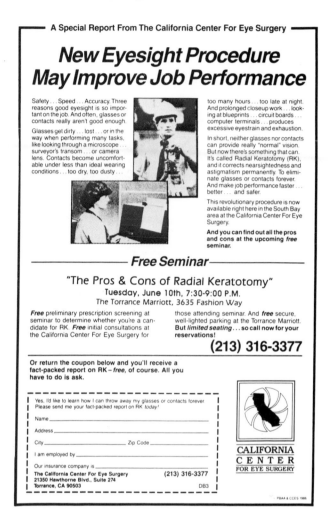

A Special Report From The California Center For Eye Surgery

New Eyesight Procedure May Improve Job Performance

Safety... Speed... Accuracy. Three reasons good eyesight is so important on the job. And often, glasses or contacts really aren't good enough.

Glasses get dirty... lost... or in the way when performing many tasks, like looking through a microscope... surveyor's transom... or camera lens. Contacts become uncomfortable under less than ideal wearing conditions... too dry, too dusty...

too many hours... too late at night. And prolonged closeup work... looking at blueprints... circuit boards... computer terminals... produces excessive eyestrain and exhaustion.

In short, neither glasses nor contacts can provide really "normal" vision. But now there's something that can. It's called Radial Keratotomy (RK), and it corrects nearsightedness and astigmatism permanently. To eliminate glasses or contacts forever. And make job performance faster... better... and safer.

This revolutionary procedure is now available right here in the South Bay area at the California Center For Eye Surgery.

And you can find out all the pros and cons at the upcoming *free* seminar.

Free Seminar

"The Pros & Cons of Radial Keratotomy"
Tuesday, June 10th, 7:30-9:00 P.M.
The Torrance Marriott, 3635 Fashion Way

Free preliminary prescription screening at seminar to determine whether you're a candidate for RK. *Free* initial consultations at the California Center For Eye Surgery for

those attending seminar. And *free* secure, well-lighted parking at the Torrance Marriott. But *limited seating*... so call now for your reservations!

(213) 316-3377

Or return the coupon below and you'll receive a fact-packed report on RK – *free*, of course. All you have to do is ask.

Yes, I'd like to learn how I can throw away my glasses or contacts forever. Please send me your fact-packed report on RK *today!*

Name _____
Address _____
City _____ Zip Code _____
I am employed by _____
Our insurance company is _____
The California Center For Eye Surgery   (213) 316-3377
21350 Hawthorne Blvd., Suite 274
Torrance, CA 90503   DB3

CALIFORNIA CENTER FOR EYE SURGERY

PBAA & CCES 1986

FIG 13–2.

☐ COPY THAT COMMANDS

Ad copy that directs the reader to take action ("Call today," "Don't put off telephoning for an appointment right now,") is often criticized as infantile and insulting. Actually, that's irrelevant—because it works.

Ad pros call it the "call to action," and no pro would ever create an ad without including one. Don't let criticism dissuade you from using command copy. The people who don't like it are usually those who won't respond regardless of the tone of the ad. Or maybe it's your office staff who knows nothing about marketing.

Response tests have repeatedly shown that, by far, commands

produce the best results. Moreover they work with just the people who count—the 1% to 5% of the readers who do respond.

☐ BEWARE OF CANNED ADS

Premade ads bought from an ad service only promote the profession. Since they're canned, they can't differentiate you from your competitors in the same specialty. This means that you're paying for an ad that'll convince prospective patients that any old competitor in your profession will do.

When They Work—Off-the-shelf ads can work when they promote a new service that most practitioners don't offer but you do. In this case, the ad must mention that the service has only limited availability.

Otherwise, stick with ad strategies that differentiate you from a sea of look-alikes.

And don't make the same mistake when you create an ad or have one done for you. You don't need to promote your specialty. You need to promote yourself and your own practice. When you spend your money, tell those prospective patients why they should come to *you* rather than someone else. For bigger personal practice growth, leave promotion of your profession to your professional association.

☐ ELEVEN WAYS TO WRITE COPY THAT GETS RESULTS

Year after year people make the same mistakes in promotion and advertising copy. The pointers that follow are particularly appropriate to keep in mind when creating a direct mail package, but they should also be followed in other promotions and advertising. You can avoid the most common and costly blunders by following these proven tips:

1. *Write in simple, colorful language.* Use short paragraphs and short words. Sixty percent of this article is short words—five letters or less. Strive for at least 65% to 76%. Keep it over 50% unless you're writing to Ph.D's. Make your sentences and paragraphs breezy. Ignore good grammar when you have a good reason. Keep the flow going: Start paragraphs with and, but, however. Use the freshest concepts and the most colorful language you can without disturbing the flow. Use "hot" words: free, new, emergency, now, secret, easy, save, guarantee, today. And the hottest word of all: you.

2. *Write lots of headlines.* Since 80% of all readers read only an ad's headline but then don't bother reading the body copy, it's the most

important part of your ad. If you don't sell in the headline, you're throwing away four fifths of your budget. Work your hardest here. As the major element in capturing attention, your headline must set forth the theme, concept, or main appeal succinctly. How? Try one of these approaches: State an advantageous claim, good advice, or news. In professional services, these are the most powerful. Always think up 10 to 100 possible headlines. Select three or four of the best based on your own and the opinion of others. Play with those for awhile, and then boil them down to one. You'll produce better headlines.

3. *Drop the warm-ups.* Get to the point at once. You'll almost destroy your direct mail letter or the ad by starting off, "You know medical expenses today have grown...."

4. *Stand out.* Separate yourself from your competition as clearly as you can. Or make your appeal uniquely urgent and important. Discover, isolate and dramatize all the reasons to come to you, not someone else. Build your entire direct mail package or ad around those reasons.

5. *Sell benefits, not features.* People don't buy products or services, they buy advantages. Service: health care. Benefits: freedom from worry, pain, illness. Talk about benefits. Be humble enough to realize that no one would give two cents for any of your service features —they're only interested in them for the benefits they give. People will pay thousands for the benefits they want.

6. *Learn to give.* Most practitioners think of their ad strictly as a device to gain new patients. Yet the readers you're addressing also want to gain something. So to succeed, as you write, adopt a giving attitude to satisfy the needs of those prospective patients. Beyond what you offer in services, you must learn to give them something immediately in the ad or direct mail letter: news, tips, interesting stories, giveaway items, and so on.

7. *Use testimonials.* They're proof that you're as good as you say you are and that you can do what you say you can. Have a successful case describe the circumstances and how he or she feels about you and your abilities. It's called credibility and you can't do a successful promotion without it. (Check your state guidelines first for any restrictions.)

8. *Money-back guarantees.* Whatever you're offering, consider including a money-back guarantee. It's a critical factor in getting someone to trust a practitioner they don't know. Or never heard of.

9. *Ask for action.* It's amazing how often otherwise good copy never gets around to asking the reader for a response. It's as simple as this: if you don't ask for action, telling them to call for an appointment, for example, you probably won't get it.

10. Budget your time. Devote about a third of your writing time to the lead elements: headline, subheads, teaser (the line on the front of the envelope), and the opening paragraph.

11. Use specialists. If you aren't experienced in direct mail writing especially, hire a specialist. Do not go to a general advertising agency. Find an experienced direct response agency with a proven track record.

REFERENCES

1. Klaus G: *Marketing By Objective* (audio cassette). 1981, Institute for Advanced Planning (256 S. La Cienega Blvd, Beverly Hills, CA 90211).
2. Perlmutter JH: *A Book of Lists for the Education Editor.* Glassboro, NJ, EDPRESS, 1984, p 121.
3. Byrne AJ, quoted in "Managing While Marketing," in *Boardroom Reports,* March 15, 1984, p 3 (500 Fifth Avenue, New York, NY).

■ CHAPTER 14
More Secrets Of The Best Promotion

☐ GREAT TYPOGRAPHY

It would seem that once you've come up with the right message for your promotional material, that just about takes care of everything, right? Not quite. In fact, all the other considerations that must be taken into account—the type to use, the kind of illustration, how large it should be—have quite an impact on the success of a marketing piece.

For example, consider typography—the typefaces you use as well as the overall appearance of the page. Great typography is pleasant looking, enticing, and clear. It helps people read your copy. Bad typography prevents reading. Let's look at some of the pointers to create good typography.

- A subhead (that's a line or two of copy that appears between the headline and the body copy) heightens the reader's appetite. It tempts and hints at what to expect.
- Body copy started with an oversized first letter (called a drop initial) is read by 13% more people.
- In long copy, after 3 or 4 in. of text, insert a subhead to break up that grey type and to keep the reader marching along. The subhead should pose a question or otherwise excite curiosity about what's to come.
- Keep paragraphs short.
- Set key paragraphs in **boldface** or *italic*.
- Use other devices such as arrows, bullets, asterisks, and margin marks to help the reader get into the paragraph. Use them sparingly, but use them when needed to draw attention.

- A line of space between paragraphs increases readership by 12%.
- White on black reversed-out body type destroys readership. Avoid it.

☐ TYPEFACES MAKE YOUR IMAGE

In promotion, including *Yellow Pages*, the typeface you use will increase or decrease the effectiveness of the piece. How? The right typeface will heighten importance, soften an edge, and increase your image of professionalism. The wrong typeface will make the ad look as if it's screeching "Bargain Basement Sale!" Since the typeface always affects the perception of the message, practitioners should use characters that deliver more character.

Typeface Guidelines—Most designers of ads could improve the image the ad conveys by increasing the sense of professionalism, dignity, or friendliness while avoiding any hint of a retail look.

To be typecast as the trustworthy cornerstone of society or bulwark of the establishment, use:

Times Roman (English)

Goudy Bold

Caslon 74 Small Caps

Baskerville (Baskerline)

Want to be friendly but professional? Try:

Souvenir Medium

Bookman Regular

For more friendliness yet, for example, if you have anything to do with children, use:

Cooper Black

For that progressive, forward-thinking look, try:

Avant Garde Medium

Eras Book

All business, no nonsense? Try the typeface many corporations use:

Helvetica

If the message is beauty, pick a pretty face. Consider:

Goudy Old Style

GASLON 451 ITALIC SWASH GAPS

Type tips:

- For heightened importance, increase the size of the letters. This works for either the headline or the body copy.
- Don't use more than two or three different typefaces in an ad. More than three causes an unpleasant appearance—as disjointed as these pages look. If more than three are crowded on the page, the piece will look like a used-car advertisement.
- Stick with easy-to-read faces. Avoid Bank Script, Engravers Old English, and other overly intricate faces that cause one's eyes to slow down while deciphering it and then perhaps stop reading altogether.
- Also steer clear of extralight faces such as Avant Garde Extra Light or Eras Light because they won't reproduce well in the poor printing of newspapers and the *Yellow Pages*.

Sticking with traditional good taste in typefaces will make your ad the class act.

☐ NO SMALL TYPE

Fully 94% of people over 60 years old report difficulty reading because of small print or poor contrast. More surprising, *56%* of those in their 30s and 45% of those in their 20s have the same complaint.

Suggestion: Generally, use no type less than 10 points in size. To give you an idea of relative size, the type you're reading in this book is set in 10-point type. Contrast is also important. Don't let your creative director get carried away. Type that will appear on colored or gray paper or over a photograph needs to be enlarged and bolder to compensate for the poor contrast. Don't make it hard for your audience to read what you have to say.

☐ POWERFUL HEADLINES

As was explained in the last chapter, 80% of all readers read only an ad's headline but don't bother reading the body copy. So the headline is the most important part of your ad. If you don't sell in the headline, you're throwing away four fifths of your budget. Work your hardest here.

As the major element in capturing attention, your headline must set forth the theme, concept, or main appeal succinctly. How? It was suggested that you try one of these approaches: State an advantageous claim, good advice, or news. In professional services, these are the most powerful.

Headline Type—The headline should be powerful, benefit-oriented, readable, and understandable. To make it readable, consider how it's typeset. In all advertising, it's not only what you say, but how it looks. This is especially true in headlines. It means style as well as readability.

So when you select headline type, have it set with initial caps and lower case for the remainder of each word. Dozens of advertising studies show that a combination of upper and lower cases enhances readership. All caps in a headline kill it.

Headline Size—The size of the headline affects readers' perceptions of the price and quality of service and therefore it influences the kind of people who respond to the ad. Some of the specific research findings[1] are as follows:

- People reading ads with larger headlines felt that meant larger discounts and lower prices *even when the ad provided no price or discount information.* Caution: The larger headlines also brought perceptions of lower quality, with traditional rather than state-of-the-art technology.
- The larger headlines also prompted people to feel that the advertiser was aiming at middle-class rather than a more up-scale audience.

What to Do—Use larger size headlines to stimulate greater attention, but include in the ad specific information about the quality of your services.

☐ AVOIDING THE AMATEUR BROCHURE

If you're not quite a pro in the brochure field but must prepare one or supervise a designer with limited experience, consider these tips:[2]

- Be guided by the principle of simplicity. Complex techniques often lose their effectiveness unless handled by a top-flight professional. And complexity causes production problems.
- Use body copy in type no smaller than 8 point and no larger than 12 point. The width of the columns of type shouldn't exceed 52 characters. Each of these parameters improves readability.
- Avoid the vertical word approach. Letters stacked in totem-pole fashion or in columns that are too thin don't work. They're too hard to read.
- Don't get cutesy in typefaces, either. Type that looks like candy canes should be saved for your office holiday party announcement. Don't use it on promotional materials that affect the health of your practice. Save the Gothic typefaces for wedding invitations. As explained previously in this chapter, ornate and other hard-to-read type styles detract from the message.
- Photos are a good idea as long as they're good ones that measure up to professional standards. Use no photographs rather than resort to poor shots.
- Insert a spot second color in the brochure sparingly. Overusing a second color is usually the mark of a novice. When in doubt, insist on seeing a color mock-up of the page so you have a very good idea of what it will look like and can see whether or not the second color is overdone.
- Don't overuse boxes and rules. Boxes (lines that surround and set off some copy) and rules (lines) can be very effective graphic devices to catch the reader's eye. But, here again, novice designers have a habit of being heavy handed with them. When you do use them, use lighter rules and smaller boxes than you originally feel would be right.
- Avoid tricky folds. If they don't work, readers won't forgive you.

Remember: Keep it simple.

☐ PHOTOGRAPHY VS. ILLUSTRATION

Ask any *successful* ad agency art director whether photographs or illustrations will make your point better, and 90% of them will say photographs without hesitating a nanosecond. Why? Because prospects can visualize more clearly and more immediately with photos. That means more powerfully. (Remember: We're interested in results, not art awards.)

The Place for Illustrations—There are some instances where an illustration makes sense:

- When it's not possible to take a photo.
- When you want to show an image that a two-dimensional photograph can't capture.

Otherwise, stick to the proven pathway. Here are the experts' photo tips for your brochures, mailers, and ads:

- Shoot close-ups and fill the photo frame with the image. This is a modern technique that makes the photo and the practice look and feel up-to-date.
- Show "after" shots. People are interested in what you can produce. Whenever appropriate, use both before-and-after shots. In a study of 70 advertising campaigns whose sales results were known, The Gallup Organization didn't find a single before-and-after campaign that failed to increase sales. If both before-and-after shots aren't possible, use the after shot alone to communicate results.
- Shoot black and white. Even in a two- or three-color brochure, black-and-white photos will do well when printed on a glossy coated paper and save you enormous full-color printing costs.
- For the *Yellow* and *Silver Pages*, have the photographs to be used in those ads printed with higher than normal contrast. With the poor printing standards of those books, subtleties are lost.

☐ HOW TO TAKE A PUBLICITY PHOTO

As long as we're discussing photography, let's talk publicity photos. Sooner or later you'll need one. If you promote at all, a publicity photo is a must—whether for a press release, press kit, practice brochure, business card, or an ad in the newspaper or *Yellow Pages*.

Your photograph helps prospects "see" what they're buying *before* they buy. And if the photo creates that solid "Dr. Welby" or "Trapper John" feeling, it's worth a lot more than a thousand words.

Guidelines—This is too important a shoot to leave to home experimentation. A professional photographer is a must. He or she will pose, light, and shoot you in ways you never thought of to put your best smile forward. The following are the techniques a pro is concerned with. If your photographer doesn't demonstrate such a concern, reconsider your choice.

- Men should wear a solid dark—but not black—suit, white shirt, and dark tie against a light background. Women should wear a solid dark suit with a light blouse against a light background. Or wear your white practice coat and shoot against a contrasting background. The contrast exudes strength. Avoid all patterns. Checks, plaids, polka dots, or big stripes, either on your clothes or the background, will distract from you. Avoid black suits because they're so dark and become an area of flat black lacking detail and dimension.
- Have the photographer shoot both color and black and white. You'll have a need for both over time.
- Have multiple poses taken: just your head and shoulders; from the waist up and leaning forward while sitting; sitting on the corner of a desk with both hands on one thigh; sitting behind a desk; and variations of each of these poses. The fewer the props, the better. That includes your latest office gizmo. No props are preferred since they too distract from the most important subject—you.
- *Smile.* It reassures your prospective patients that everything's going to turn out okay.
- *Relax.* If you're feeling stiff, you'll project it. Have the photographer shoot a few shots just to relax you. You need to be loose, so joke, laugh—do whatever, and enjoy yourself. Otherwise, you'll look like a mortician.
- Have the photographer use lighting to create depth in your face. A three-quarter angle flood will cast enough soft shadow to give your face character. Also diffuse all background shadows, and make sure nothing casts a shadow on you.
- Have the photographer shoot and print in higher than normal contrast. It's a stronger photo and will reproduce better

on paper, again, especially with the inexpensive printing
used in phone directories.

■ If the photos on the proof sheet aren't perfect, that isn't necessarily reason to worry. The photographer can crop, i.e.,
chop off, part of the photograph or have it airbrushed. Airbrushing can take care of facial and other blemishes or virtually anything else unwanted in the print. But if the
problem isn't one that can be corrected with cropping or airbrushing—for example, if you don't look confident in the
shot—then it's time to start over.

Suggestion—Give your photographer a copy of this article just to
double check. It's your insurance policy for those photographers who
don't specialize in portraits.

One last directive: Tell your photographer, "Above all, make me
look trustworthy."

☐ COMPUTERIZED AD ANALYSES

Traditionally, advertising researchers have had to second-guess
how readers would respond to their ads. Or they've buttonholed
people in a market sample and hoped that those individuals were
giving their honest reactions.

That imprecision wasn't good enough for Elliot Young, president
of Perception Research Services (PRS).[3] Young uses an innovative
eye-tracking technique that records the part of an ad a person is
viewing. An invisible infrared beam is focused on the subject's pupil.
Thirty times a second the beam discerns which particular word or
other part of an ad the subject is looking at, as well as how long he
or she looked at it.

Young's computers can even play back a viewing session, showing exactly how a subject's eyes scanned—or missed—part of an ad.

Findings—Eye-tracking studies show that 43% of readers never even
see the advertiser's name on the average ad. And that translates to
$800 million annually lost in wasted advertising.

PRS studies have also documented the following results:

1. Ad design: When it comes to visuals (illustrations or photographs), people spend time looking at the pictures and may even miss
the product or service, the copy, or the name of the advertiser. The
average person spends 65% of his or her ad-viewing time on the
visuals. Only 35% is spent on copy. So make sure your visuals relate

directly to your service and that they're not there just for attention-stopping purposes. Yes, they should grab attention, but the reader may not look beyond them.

2. Size of ads: Spreads (advertisements that run across two facing pages) have 60% more stopping power than a single-page ad. While 9% of readers miss single-page ads, no one misses a spread. One other benefit: In spreads, 71% see the advertiser's name; in single-page ads, only 62% do. The drawback, of course, is the cost. Spreads usually cost twice as much as a single-page ad. When it comes to the benefits of a full-page ad vs. a partial-page ad, the results are conclusive. The average single-page ad generates 181% more involvement than the partial page advertisement. Color has the advantage of boosting stopping power 13 percentage points over black and white in newspapers and magazines. So if the cost is greater than that increase in response, pass on color and save.

3. Editorial environment: The placement of an ad significantly affects its success. An ad appearing opposite strong editorial matter with good visuals elicits less response than an ad appearing opposite uninteresting editorial matter. So you want your ad to border the boring. Ads may also be hurt by facing ads. For example, professional practice ads on facing pages compete with each other to the disadvantage of both.

☐ THE 10-SECOND PRETEST

Take your completed print ad and find out if it will do what you want it to do *before* you spend money in the media.

Show it to friends, associates, patients, anyone who'll look at it. But have them glance at it for *only 10 seconds*. Ask them to describe the message the ad puts across. If it matches your original objective, you have an effective ad.

If not, regardless of how beautiful you think the ad is, send your copywriter and artist back to the drawing board. Make sure that when they create an ad, they remember what the prime objective is—what you want the readers to remember and what action you want them to take. Say this in your headline, in the photograph or illustration, and in the body copy.

REFERENCES

1. Billizzi JA, Hite RE: The effects of sale headline size and position on perceived discount levels and other perceptual measures. *Communica-*

tions Briefings, October 1985, p 9 (P. O. Box 587, Glassboro, NJ 08028).

2. Pickens JE: *The Copy to Press Handbook.* New York, John Wiley & Sons, 1983.

3. Young E: Eye tracking studies open eyes. *Communications Briefings,* October 1984, p 3 (P. O. Box 587, Glassboro, NJ 08028).

■ PART 3 The Execution: Media Specifics

■ CHAPTER 15
The *Yellow Pages*: Your Second Best Return On Investment

The answer to that question is not just yes, it's a resounding yes! According to a Ruben Donnelly study, listings for professionals were among the most used of all.

The average *Yellow Pages* directory contains over 4,900 headings. Here's how professionals stack up within the top 100 *Yellow Pages* headings in terms of public usage:

CATEGORY	RANK
Attorneys	8
Physicians and surgeons (MDs)	23
Dentists	32
Optometrists	81

The majority of the top 100 headings are for personal services, rather than for retailers selling products as one might think. And the top three categories? Insurance ranked number one, restaurants were second, and real estate listings came in third.

Little wonder then that practitioners are increasingly turning to the *Yellow Pages* to reach their prospects. The number of *Yellow Pages* ads for professional services has been growing by leaps and bounds. According to Market Data Retrieval in Westport, Conn, one of the country's largest compilers of lists of professionals taken from telephone directories, professionals are placing *Yellow Pages* ads as never before. In one 12-month period—between August 1983 and August 1984—the number of physicians who used directory display advertisements grew by 13.7%. Other professionals are likewise increasing their *Yellow Pages* advertising dramatically. And there's evidence that such display ads have jumped even more since that time.

Is it Dignified and Professional?—Yes and no. It's not if you put in the typical retail *Yellow Pages* ad that makes you look like a snake oil salesperson. But certainly if it creates a professional image, it will be dignified just as a Mercedes or Jaguar ad is. It's not the media that determines your image, but what you put in it.

☐ WHO NEEDS TO BE IN THE *YELLOW PAGES*

Practically all private, primary care physicians can benefit from *Yellow Pages* display ads. That's also true for those specialties that prospective patients now seek out on their own. But for some practitioners, the *Yellow Pages* directory is more crucial than for others. Who are they?

Those practitioners who are needed by their patients *only on occasion* should think twice before dismissing this medium. When you want to reach new patients looking for a practitioner in your field, the *Yellow Pages* is the only place where they can find your message 365 days a year. That's not the case with public relations, speeches, articles, direct mail, or ads in newspapers, magazines, radio or television. That, plus the fact that the public's been shopping here for some 80 years makes that directory perfect for reaching new patients.

Results—One Wisconsin OB/GYN reports that 14% of his last year's patients came either from his *Yellow Pages* ad or as referrals from women who originally came in because of that ad. "That's a sizable change compared to 2 years ago when we totally relied on referrals from professionals and word of mouth."

☐ AD ANALYSIS: POPPING OFF THE PAGE

If your ad doesn't get noticed, the response will be too small for you to notice. In the classically designed ad in Figure 15-1, the big visual accomplishes two purposes. One, it grabs attention away from all the other display ads in the directory. And two, the friendly, competent-looking doctor reassures the prospective patient that in his hands, everything's all right. Notice the very modern mezzo screen that the art director used on the photo to make it the most unusual and noticeable one in the book. That boosts response. For an idea of how noticeable this ad is, put it next to the ads in your *Yellow Pages* section, and compare.

The suprahead (at the top of the ad and above the headline), quickly targets the market that is sought. The headline talks powerfully of the doctor's long list of accomplishments. The credentials set off with bullets prove the headline's claims. And the quote adds the dimension of great caring.

Add the benefit of accepting Medicare assignments, set the whole ad in a solid, serif typeface, and you've got an impressive, professional, and profitable *Yellow Pages* presence.

☐ *YELLOW PAGES:* ONE OF THE BEST BANGS FOR YOUR BUCK

Physicians often ask, "Why would someone pick a practitioner from the *Yellow Pages?*" Yet those professionals who invest in *Yellow Pages* advertising answer that whatever the reason, the fact remains that people do turn to the *Yellow Pages*—in droves. They've found that advertising can easily deliver a 1000% return on investment (ROI).

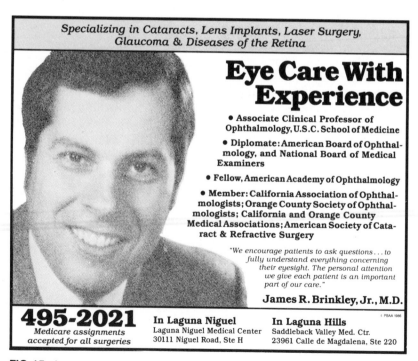

FIG 15–1.

It's hard to find an investment of any kind where the risk is so low with returns that high.

Low Risk—The risk is low for two reasons. The first has to do with the large case size, which most practitioners tend to underestimate, of the average new patient during their first year with you. The experience of *The Practice Builder* is that professionals tend to underestimate average income per new patient over the first year by 20% to 30%.

Over the life of that new patient, the case size can be enormous. For example, the mean expenditure per pediatric patient over the first 18 years exceeds $13,000. That's a lot of inoculations and runny noses—and nothing to sneeze at. With such a large case size, even low response rates mean big payoffs.

The second reason for the low risk comes from the lack of *sophisticated* competition in the *Yellow Pages*. Almost everyone advertising there takes advantage of the free design work available from the directory's art department. The results: the ad looks like that for a tire store; the marketing strategies are nonexistent.

But when a sophisticated ad appears that says the right message with the right graphics, it stands alone, even in a crowded directory. The quality of your ads has a much greater impact on your bottom line than the quantity of your competitors.

Potential, Not Panacea—The returns that a *Yellow Pages* ad can deliver aren't guaranteed. Will your ad pay? The answer is a qualified yes. Yes, if the position or placement is right; yes, if the headline and copy are right; and yes, if the graphics grab the reader.

Beware: If the *Yellow Pages* competition increases significantly and your response dips, don't discontinue your *Yellow Pages* promotion. Instead, improve your *Yellow Pages* strategies to respond to the new competition, and continue close tracking. If after those adjustments, your results don't respond and you're running at a loss from the *Yellow Pages*, the competition may have sliced up the pie too thinly. In that case, other promotional avenues may now deserve your dollars more. But don't discontinue if you're at breakeven. Because of the potential return, making more adjustments is the smarter move.

THREE WINNING *YELLOW PAGES* STRATEGIES: POSITION, POSITION, POSITION

A *Yellow Pages* ad ranks second only to your outdoor office sign in its ability to generate big income compared to its cost. And because the return can be so large, it almost always pays to spend what you need to improve results. But what's the best way to do this?

With *Yellow Pages* ads, *position is 80%* of the success equation. Reason: People shop from the front to the back of the 'A' section, starting with the display ads. And they stop looking seriously as soon as they find a message they like.

Winning Strategy—The *Yellow Pages* determines the position of the ads within each section by size with the largest first. (Among the same-sized ads, forward position usually goes to advertisers with more seniority. But in a small number of directories, it's done by alphabetical order. Check your book to see which method is used.) So the bigger the ad you buy, the better its position. That translates into more business for you. Buy big to gain the most forward position of the section to capture the lion's share of prospective patients.

To find out exactly how big to buy, in your section of the current directory circle all the display ads for those with offices within 3 to 5 miles of yours. These are your main competitors. Buy an ad that's one size larger than the biggest one to gain the premier position. At minimum, have an ad that's as big as those of your competitors.

Two Caveats—One of the caveats applies in those rare directories that have a page of in-columns ads, called "trademarks," preceding the display ads. In this case you still buy for position but now it's determined alphabetically rather than by size. If your last—or first—name begins with "A", place a large in-column ad. By adding color, you're sure to be noticed. End result: lower bills and better results than the display ads that follow the in-column ads.

Unless the in-column ads precede the display ads, they only serve two purposes. First, they satisfy the timid professional concerned about building his or her practice but still afraid that display advertising will be frowned on by colleagues. And second, they make money for the *Yellow Pages*, but not necessarily for the practitioner. The in-column strategy, unless they appear before display ads, is to take the free listing only and place your resources in a good display advertisement.

Few Competitors—The second caveat applies when there's little or no competition in the display ads. Here, buy small since you'll be the only one or one of few. But it can be difficult to be the first.

For example, psychiatrist B.C. of Arkansas called *The Practice Builder* advisory hotline with that troubling situation. "What do I do if no one in my profession has ever had a *Yellow Pages* ad before and it's considered almost unethical?"

☐ What To Spend In The White Pages

Nothing. People shop in the *Yellow Pages*, not the white. So take the free listing, and don't listen to the rep trying to convince you to spend more.

Fewer and fewer directories around the country have no display ads in the "physicians and surgeons" section. Those that remain might be in areas where there are so few practitioners that none have felt the need to run an ad. Or they're in places where members of the local society have secretly agreed that no member should place an individual ad. Yet that agreement is in violation of Federal Trade Commission guidelines as a restraint of trade. The society had better hope there's no whistle-blower around.

Still, most professionals don't want to break the *Yellow Pages* barrier. If you're the first, you'll be leading the charge on a new frontier, and you risk being shot full of arrows from disapproving colleagues. (Or is "competitors" a more accurate term?) They'll disapprove because they fear being hurt financially yet are envious of your courage.

But if you decide to be that frontier marketer, you'll have much consolation. Even though shot full of arrows, you'll have gained enough new patients to afford the best medical attention available. And once the wounds have healed, invariably, others will start display advertising also. The next year, two or three more ads will appear. Then the flood gates will open.

If you face a virgin *Yellow Pages* section, your decison is whether to be first or to be a follower later because eventually someone will break ranks. The rewards are simply too great to stop it from happening sooner or later.

Results—Northeast ophthalmologist C.P. looked to expand his caseload of cataract surgeries. Starting off, he went with a 1-in. *Yellow Pages* in-column bold listing. The results were as shallow as the ad. In year two, he tested a 1-column × 2 1/2-in. display ad. The year's cost of $636 for the ad resulted in eight cataract patients. In year 3, he escalated to a quarter-page ad (2-columns × 5-in.) and received 14 surgeries.

"Being the first ophthalmologist with a display ad obviously helped. But also in this case, the bigger the ad, the better the results."

☐ WHICH DIRECTORY TO CHOOSE

With so many new choices, which directory to advertise in seems like a troublesome decision. But not if you follow these guidelines:

1. Go into the big book: The main book in your area for the last 80 years does charge more because people use it more. And that means you get more response. People's habits don't change easily or quickly. They'll continue to use the big book and you'll continue to profit by being in it. Remember: Don't fixate on the expense—evaluate the return on investment only.

2. Avoid copycat books: The mere fact that a book is distributed doesn't mean that it's used. To change consumers' habit of turning to the big book would take a consistent campaign on radio and television. But few new books are willing to front that budget because they figure advertisers won't bother to track the responses they receive. So avoid the new start-ups that try to look and feel like the old and established—unless they spend for public awareness. Remember: Copycat books are cheap for a reason. Buy for results, not for cost.

3. Consider small community books: When your local big book is big—really big—and covers a large area, consider also using a small community book. But when you do, you'll need to ask new patients how they heard about you so you can track the book's effectiveness. Test for one year, and continue if profitable.

4. Test the Silver Pages: This specialty book is geared to people over 60 years of age and lists advertisers offering a senior's discount. The *Silver Pages* can work—if you target seniors, if you convey the right message, if you have the right ad position, and so on. It doesn't work for all, just as the *Yellow Pages* doesn't. So if you want to profit as America grays, test and track the *Silver Pages* for a year before renewing.

5. Test other specialty books: There are now Spanish-language directories as well as Christian, Asian, and others catering to various target groups. Each should be evaluated on its own merits, especially as to whether you are *centrally located* for most of those receiving the book. Practitioners located on the fringe of a book's area rarely do well. Again, test and evaluate.

6. Avoid organization directories: The Chamber of Commerce, Better Business Bureau, and others are all cashing in on the *Yellow Pages* craze as they search for new sources of funding. In a recent *Practice Builder* survey of 61 practitioners with an ad in an organization's directory, *none* showed a profit.

☐ AD ANALYSIS

Here's another *Yellow Pages* ad that deserves close study. The ad shown in Figure 15–2 is eye-catching, even at a glance, because of it's very clean, uncluttered look. Imagine how that airy look will set it apart from all the retail-looking ads surrounding it.

Its design is carefully constructed to convey the feeling that this practice is both friendly and very up-to-date. Both of those attributes will strongly appeal to prospective patients in this affluent area. But the design and the headline also promise "a difference"—that this practice isn't numbered among the commonplace.

That "difference" is reinforced throughout the ad. The practice's upscale location is another drawing card that is played in the supra-head. And the credentials, treatments, and services that are listed in

---

IN PALOS VERDES

It's Family Medicine With A Difference

- Over 13 years experience in the practice of medicine
- Routine & emergency care

Plus:

- Aviation medical exams (Class II & III)
- Allergy control
- Sports medicine & injury care
- Alcohol & substance abuse
- Nutritional counseling
- Personal & on-the-job injury care
- Weight control using a revolutionary real foods program

It's experienced, concerned care — with a difference.

P&AA 1986

| Open Mon, Tues,
Thurs & Fri
Insurance welcome
VISA MasterCard | **Call 377-4222**
Richard C. Keech, M.D.
Member: California Medical Association,
L.A. County Medical Association &
American Society of Clinical Pathologists | 827 Deep Valley Dr.,
Suite 207
Rolling Hills Estates |

FIG 15–2.

the ad were carefully chosen for their appeal to this market and to differentiate the practice.

Finally, notice the tag line, "It's experienced, concerned care— with a difference." As far as the ad is concerned, the big difference is style. And it works.

☐ MORE RESULTS—NO GUESSWORK

How do you test the effectiveness of different directories? Simple. Key each *Yellow Pages* ad and all other promotions in a similar manner using one of three keying systems.

Key System 1: If you have separate telephone lines available to dedicate, show one telephone number in one of the ads being tested, while each other ad lists another distinct number. Then every time the telephone rings, you know exactly which ad prompted the call.

Key System 2: Not enough lines? Use fictitious extensions. Calls asking for extension three identifies prospective patients responding to a specific ad or medium. Extension ten keys another ad or medium.

Key System 3: This is a variation on the second suggestion. One of your ads prompts readers to ask for Jane for an appointment. "Jane" is the key for ad 1; "Cory" keys 2, and so forth.

By having the desk keep a close count of the calls coming in and the new cases generated, you're in a position to analyze the effectiveness of your campaigns. Only one statistic counts—return on investment. Divide the total income generated through that source by the cost of that medium. Also interesting but not as crucial is the number and size of cases generated by each medium or ad.

This is all the data you need to test a directory or otherwise to decide whether an ad is effective.

☐ WHAT TO SAY IN THE *YELLOW PAGES*

For his *Yellow Pages* headline, psychiatrist J.L. wrote, "Therapy may be the answer you've been seeking." And family practitioner N.M. used his name as the headline. Both made crucial mistakes.

In the psychiatrist's case, he assumed he was promoting psychiatry, but any prospective patient who turned to that section had already decided to use a psychiatrist. The only question that needed to be answered was "which one?"

In the family practitioner's case, N.M. believed that his name was sufficient to interest a prospective patient to read his ad. Unfortunately, that's only true for his wife and mother—not for all those prospects unknown to him.

Essential Questions—The public brings an essential question to the *Yellow Pages*. As they begin to read your ad, they're asking themselves, "Why you?" In other words, they're asking, "What's in it for me? How do you differ from the competition? And how can you fill my needs?" Prospective patients will give you a second or two glance in which you must communicate your answer, or *they won't read the rest of the ad*. Period. Therefore put the reasons in *your headline*.

The headline must promise or imply a benefit to the reader: *fast relief, greater experience, special expertise, affordable prices, convenient hours, high technology, greater caring,* and so forth.

Location is also a strong point of differentiation. Since trading zones are relatively small, especially for services requiring repeat visits, where you're located is always important. But don't put it in the headline. Instead, put the *locale* you serve *above the headline* in smaller type. Either the name of the town, towns, or parts of the city. This highlights location and still gives you an opportunity to state another benefit in the headline.

Body Copy—Below the headline write one or two short paragraphs proving or expanding on the claim in the headline. Without substantiation, your claims lose credibility.

For the secondary benefits, create a list below the paragraphs: hours (if convenient); payment options; little-known services you provide. Now that you've convinced the reader, close out the ad with "fulfillment information"—your name, address, telephone number, and logo.

A Second Essential Question—People also need to know if they can trust you. They may not ask themselves the question consciously, but those ads that address it will always outpull those that don't. Here are the four classic ways to foster trust in a *Yellow Pages* ad.

The first is the use of a clean, professional-looking layout with a nonretail typeface. The second is through the use of educational credentials, authorships, awards, endorsements, memberships, and the like. The third is by the quality of the copywriting. If it's professional, then by implication, so are you. And fourth is by including your tasteful, professionally taken photograph.

☐ PROFESSIONAL ART MAKES THE DIFFERENCE

Does your *Yellow Pages* ad look more like one for a used car dealer? Or does it look like an award-winning ad suitable for framing, but gets no results. The former can happen from using the writers and artists provided free by the *Yellow Pages*. And the latter can be the result of using an expensive ad agency that has never created a *Yellow Pages* ad before.

Superior artwork and layout can give a *Yellow Pages* display ad the major share of attention in the directory. Results often differ by 15 to 1. Given that spread in results, it makes sense to use professional talent—especially when the monthly *Yellow Pages* bill runs $500 or more. When the ad's results can vary so dramatically, a $500 art bill becomes insignificant.

☐ INVESTING IN COLOR: IS IT WORTH IT?

The *Yellow Pages* rep tells you your ad will be noticed if you use color in it. Then later the rep mentions that it raises the price of the ad 50% to 100%. Is it worth it? Rarely. Sparkling graphics and a strong headline will attract the attention of more readers than using color in the ad. And the cost of professional graphics and copy is not only less than the cost of using color, it's a one-time cost.

There is one time when it is wise to use color in the *Yellow Pages*. When most of the display ads have been professionally produced with good graphics and copy (not those prepared by the *Yellow Pages* staff), then use color to compete for attention. However, there are few if any *Yellow Pages* in the country with sections for professional services that fit that description.

☐ *YELLOW PAGES* GIMMICKS TO AVOID AND A FEW WARNINGS

Some ideas and outfits just don't deserve your attention or your trust. Tactics such as putting your ad on a plastic cover for consumers' *Yellow Pages* directories just don't work. Here's a list of temptations and tactics to avoid when it comes to the *Yellow Pages*. So caveat emptor:

1. *Trusting the* Yellow Pages *to contact you in time:* If it happens, be thankful. With so much turnover in reps and management, expect huge cracks in their systems. If your account falls into one, you won't

be given enough warning to prepare the ad you want. Don't rely on their staff. Assume it's your responsibility, and call them now to find out their closing date if they prepare the ad and the later camera-ready closing date if you supply a finished ad to them.

2. *Peel-off stickers for the* Yellow Pages: Some entrepreneurs are trying to corner those professionals who've just opened their practice, relocated, or otherwise missed being included in the *Yellow Pages*. They want to print your name and other information on a sticker that they mail along with other stickers to homes for gluing into the *Yellow Pages* directory. The problem: People won't sit and stick in the labels. Bigger problem: If you missed the book, you're already paying for it.

3. *Talking* Yellow Pages: With this, prospects call a central number to reach an operator who gives the name and other particulars of the advertisers in this spoken directory. The problem: People are used to the printed *Yellow Pages*. To switch them over would require a megabuck advertising campaign that these start-up operations don't have.

4. *Ads by committee:* Creating *Yellow Pages* ads by a committee of partners, staff, friends, or spouses doesn't work. What comes out of committee is a bland, confusing compromise of ideas that can't convince any prospective patient of anything.

5. *Trusting the* Yellow Pages *for strategies:* Don't ask the *Yellow Pages* ad department what to put in your ad. The only thing they can tell you is what others have done—which is the blind leading the blind. Beyond that, the best they'll be able to do is repeat the company line—that you should include who, what, where, when. Unfortunately, these aren't strategies that answer the questions in prospective patients minds about what distinquishes you from other physicians and whether you're trustworthy.

PRETEST AVOIDS MISTAKES

Ever have a *Yellow Pages* ad that you thought would be the best in the book, but when it was published, it looked all wrong and out of place? This isn't an uncommon situation for those who've never put together a directory ad before.

The Problem—The ad can't be created in a vacuum. The environment in which it will appear should be considered. Ask yourself, how does the ad compare to others? How would a prospective patient react to yours while glancing at it and the others in the same section?

The Solution—To answer those questions, you need to pretest the

effectiveness of your ad. Take a full-size mock-up of your ad, pho-
tocopy it onto yellow paper, and paste the copy into last year's *Yellow
Pages* in the section where it will appear. Then leaf through that section
as a prospective patient would. Have others do the same. Does the
ad fit well into the book and still pop out at you in a pleasing and
interesting way? Or does it pop out because it looks so out of place?
Is it convincing, given the competition?

   If you and the others react negatively, it's time to start over at
square one with a new creative or artistic strategy *now*. Remember:
If you don't pretest, you're going to be stuck with an unsatisfactory
ad for the next 365 days.

■ CHAPTER 16
Direct Mail Directives: The How-To's Of A 400% Return In 90 Days

☐ WHY DIRECT MAIL?

Often cited in the business as a marketing legend, Bob Stone[1] points to direct mail as the one truly unique medium, especially for professionals. With the exceptions of outdoor office signs and *Yellow Pages*, direct mail will usually produce the highest percentage of response. And that means the highest percentage of profits. Why? Three reasons—targetability, deliverability, and affordability.

Targetability—You can select a mailing list that zeros in on a certain type of person by age, income, household size, or other characteristics. And you can make your message a personal one by using a computer-generated letter that addresses each individual by name. And the letter can use copy focused directly on the characteristics that distinguish the specific lists you use.

Best of all, you can mail to just the geographic area you choose, without waste. No other medium, not radio, television, magazines, or newspapers affords that targetability. That's efficiency.

Deliverability—Direct mail is free of the big problems that plague other media. Your newspaper ad may reach your prospective patients—if they read the paper that day, if they turn to the page where your ad appears, and if they read the ad itself. Lots of ifs. Magazines are the same, while television and radio present similar situations.

But direct mail gets delivered. With your message in your prospect's hands, your only challenge is to interest them enough to open and read the letter. Essentially, direct mail removes many of the ifs.

Affordability—Mail as few or as many as you like, as often as you can afford. Flexibility like that makes direct mail affordable. And since the response is immediate, the expense of repetition needed with other media can be cut down or avoided.

Cost? In the area of $200 to $500 per 1,000 pieces mailed. Plus development costs of $500 on the low side to $5,000 on the high side depending on the package configuration.

☐ HOW TO DO GREAT DIRECT MAIL

Illinois internist R.D. mailed 10,000 direct mail pieces to addresses within a 3-mile radius of his office. He received 134 calls, completed treatment on 54 who spent an average of $612 each for a total of $33,748—all in 90 days time. Very impressive.

So is the case of California physician T.B. She mailed 6,000 pieces to homeowners within a 5-mile radius who had homes valued in excess of $100,000. Seven people called, four made appointments. Only two kept them and spent money. Total income: $368. Total loss: $2,152.

What do these cases illustrate? The first case points up that direct mail can be highly profitable. The second demonstrates that it's also highly risky. In fact, direct mail is by far the most difficult of all promotions to create.

The reason is that unlike other media, direct mail has an entire body of techniques that must be woven throughout the material, or you simply don't generate phone calls. No if, ands, or buts. In addition, you must marry these techniques to the optimal strategies for promoting and differentiating your practice. Two sets of strategies mean twice as many ways to make a mistake. And just one mistake can doom a project.

Add to this the problem that most advertising people don't really know direct mail techniques because they've never studied them and they don't use them every day. On top of that, few creative people know both direct mail and your profession's strategies. If direct mail is hard for pros, it's really hard for an individual practitioner.

So all but the simplest direct mail is best left to the right pros, unless you prefer to learn the expensive way. Okay to do yourself: Cooperative coupons, repetitive new resident mailings consisting of a benefit-oriented letter and welcoming certificate, or quarterly mailings to your existing patients. Best left to pros: Cold prospecting mailings to the general public or specific markets with whom you've had no previous contact.

However, it certainly doesn't hurt to understand the following techniques and strategies. You'll be better able to select proper direct mail talent for the tough jobs as well as to create your own promotional pieces, where appropriate.

Direct Response vs. Name Recognition—Direct mail becomes direct response by virtue of the offer it contains. Without an offer, the 1% response rate that's traditionally bandied about will be much, much lower. And when the pieces go out with an offer, response comes in now, not later. But as soon as the offer is over within a few weeks of mailing, response nosedives. So you best be back in the mail again to an entirely new list of prospective patients. You shouldn't remail to the first group until it's been left fallow for at least 90 days.

But there's also another strategy for direct mail called name recognition mailing. In this case, there's no offer, just strong non-monetary reasons to respond. However, like other nondirect response, you must have repetition to make it work. That means mailing now, then in 30 days, then 90 days, and at 90-day intervals after that.

Many physicians and other professionals don't like the idea of making an offer, which is fine. But one mailing in a name recognition promotion is a waste of money. Remember the required rule of repetition if you decide to play this game. And with repetition, response builds slowly. So don't expect a quick payback.

However, most practitioners don't have the budget or stomach lining to wait. They need to see big dollars come in immediately. Therefore, many practitioners will make direct response mailings one right after another, each with a different offer. This gives a quick response, time after time, and it also nicely builds recognition of your name over time. You get both the numbers and the name.

Direct Mail Techniques— For cold prospect mailings where you've had no previous contact with the recipient, self-mailers tend to give greater response than envelope mailings. Direct mail wisdom usually argues the opposite, but *The Practice Builder's* controlled tests point to self-mailers as the best vehicles in promoting professional services. If you use an offer, print, and insert it as a separate coupon. It raises responses if it's separate rather than a perforated panel.

Offers must look like offers. Use heavy borders, big headlines, attention-grabbing graphics. If they don't see the offer, you won't see the response.

In 99% of these mailings, you'll mail them bulk rate to save money. It now costs 10.1 cents for carrier route presorted mail and up to 12.5 cents for regular third class. First class rarely buys you anything. So use a preprinted indicia (postal permit) since it's the cheapest way to affix postage. If your mailing is intended to look personal, send it in an envelope that is then postage metered or has a precanceled third-class bulk rate stamp. These are both slightly more expensive to process but reinforce the desired feeling.

On large mailings, always use a letter shop or mailing service. Your staff simply can't or won't get it out the door on time. A letter shop will mail it inexpensively for you within 1 to 3 days. Don't economize here.

The Right Lists—In cold prospect mailings, it's fine to use labels addressed to "resident." Since it's obviously advertising, no addressee names are required as in more personalized mailings. But do make sure when mailing to apartment renters or condo owners that their unit numbers are on the label. Otherwise, the postal carrier just dumps them in the bottom communal bin as a "take one." Your piece won't make it into the individual mailbox.

Caution dictates mailing only 4,000 or 5,000 of a new direct mail package to start. This allows you to see how well the package and list work and limits your exposure before investing in a larger mailing. It also permits you to gauge the speed of response and intelligently schedule your next mail drop. In this way, you don't overload the office and make new patients wait 4 weeks to see you.

Close to Home—The smart mailer first targets addresses right around the office. The closer in, the greater the response. If you track from where the respondents come, you'll know how far away from the office you can profitably mail. Mail until you break even. Then go back to the original homes to whom you mailed and start again. Wait at least 90 days between mailings to the same addresses. To keep the piece fresh for repetitive mailings, just change one or two colors to give the piece a whole new feel and keep responses up.

Costs vary but overall, this is a high risk, high gain game—the costs are commensurate with the potential return. Count on 15 to 20 cents for printing a self-mailer, 2 to 5 cents for each label, 10.1 to 12.5 cents postage, and 2 cents for each piece for the letter shop to mail them out. Total: 30 to 45 cents each. Expensive? Yes. Profitable? Highly. Risky? Uh, huh.

Great Direct Mail—Figures 16–1 through 16–6 illustrate a prime example of effective direct mail. This copyright-protected piece was created by The Practice Builder Ad Agency for a special program staffed by a psychologist-dentist team to treat dental fears. Direct mail was the medium chosen because it gave unlimited space to sell a brand-new concept. Also, there was no affordable newspaper coverage in this small suburb of a large, southwest city.

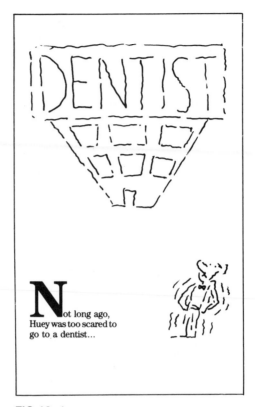

FIG 16–1.

The 3 3/4 × 6-in. piece folds out to 12 panels to unveil the story of Huey, who's been afraid of the dentist since childhood. The copy explains how Huey hasn't seen a dentist since then, but now he's heard about something new.

With each panel, Huey becomes larger, more confident. The copy identifies with his problem and explains the benefits of this new and unique program. In this way, the visuals explain and illustrate the benefits of the service. That makes it a powerful piece.

Unique Look—Smooth, convincing copy, a tantalizing cover, benefit after benefit, and superstrong visuals add up to a must-read piece. It certainly looks different than any other piece in the mailbox, and that usually means more readership and more response.

With an insert about program specifics and costs, this will also act as the office's practice brochure. It's an inexpensive way to kill two birds with one budget.

☐ HOW TO FIND THE RIGHT MAILING LIST

As direct mail becomes more prevalent among professionals, the art of selecting the right mailing list becomes more crucial. Why? There's an adage in direct mail that 40% of the package's success is due to what you say, 20% from how you say it, but *a full 40%* is determined by reaching the right people. That means finding the right list.

The Right People—The better you define who's most likely to respond, the more refined your list selection will be—and the more response you'll get. You'll also save considerable money by not mailing to every household within a 3-mile radius of your office. Define your targets using age, sex, family size, household income, religion, ethnicity, race, interests, homeowners vs. renters, age of children, whether they've responded to direct mail before, and, of course, location. Only by sharply pinpointing the characteristics of those you want most to respond can you zero in on the list you should order.

Now there's *individual* information on about 80% of the households in the country drawn from sources as varied as drivers' license files, property deeds, auto registration records, telephone books, city directories, professional and club registries, and boat and airplane ownership or operators' files.

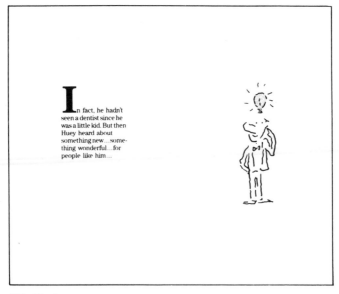

FIG 16–2.

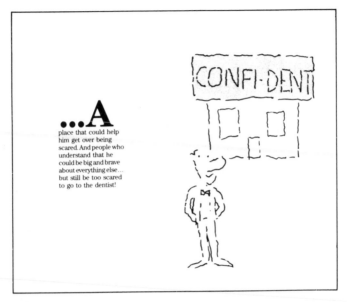

FIG 16–3.

Pinpoint Precision—And the demographic specialists have come up with computer programs that can correlate U.S. census data estimates to areas as small as a city block. Focusing in on specific neighborhoods instead of much larger zip code areas, this technology lets you examine and extract areas with a specific income range, racial/ethnic mix, even home ownership, presence of children, and age of the head of the household.

Today, taking advantage of that sophisticated computerization, practitioners can rent lists along practically any parameters. For example, income alone can be a poor selector of prime prospects. Instead, a better profile is created by a combination of income, education, and occupation. So sophisticated indices like the Social Position Index, CACI, Data Fax, and PRIZD Cluster Segmentation have been developed. Each one massages a different combination of demographics to produce a highly segmented group. Then you mail to your top groups, making your whole mailing more responsive and less costly.

Index by Neighborhood—These index selections are available for an entire zip code or postal carrier route or even a block group, but not for individual dwellings. That means you would need to mail the entire block group, carrier route, or zip code. A block group is the smallest breakdown and approximates a neighborhood consisting of about 250 residences.

For larger mailings, some list compilers will even take your patient list and analyze it to ascertain what combination of demographics you're already attracting by matching their names against their census data.

Broker Expertise—To find lists to rent, look under "mailing lists" in the *Yellow Pages* of the nearest large city. You're looking for list brokers among those listed. When you contact the list brokers, tell them who your most likely prospects are. You'll quickly discover how they'll help you define your market even more and rent you the right list. The brokers will tell you how many names fall into different categories. Some are very sophisticated while many others aren't. And beware of those who will try to rent you a list that's off base.

Lists are rented for one-time use only. For each additional mailing, you must rerent the list. Rent, don't buy or try to construct a permanent list yourself. Without a method of continual updating for relocations and deaths, the list becomes quickly outdated. That updating is the reason you rent a list, but you must check to see how often the list is cleaned. A list over 1 or 2 years old that has not been updated will contain a high percentage of undeliverable names. Look for updates within 12 months, preferably within 6 months.)

Personal Inspection—And remember to always personally inspect the list since too many expensive mailings have been ruined by the broker sending *the wrong list*. The consequence of mailing the wrong

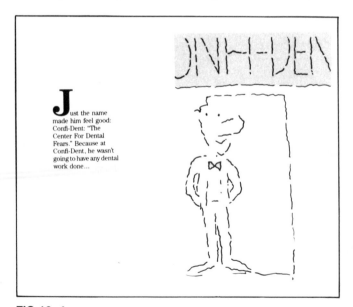

FIG 16–4.

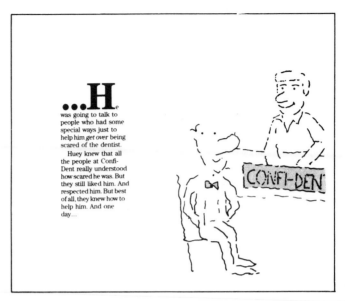

...He was going to talk to people who had some special ways just to help him *get over* being scared of the dentist.

Huey knew that all the people at Confi-Dent really understood how scared he was. But they still liked him. And respected him. But best of all, they knew how to help him. And one day...

FIG 16–5.

list is usually total loss. In one recent case, an M.D. ordered a list of people in his area only to receive a list of residents in a city 10 miles away!

So look for numerous duplicates, wrong zip codes, company names when you ordered residences, apartment numbers if you ordered homeowners. If your letter shop or agency orders the list for you, personally inspect it before you give the go-ahead to affix the labels. If you're ordering it yourself, have it sent to your office so that you can inspect it personally.

Costs—Price ranges from $20 per thousand (2 cents each) to about $50 per thousand, depending on how refined the list is. Although the list broker is employed by you, he or she is usually paid by the list owner with a percentage of the rental. You won't save that commission by renting directly from the list owner.

Because the cost of renting a mailing list makes up such a minor portion of the cost of a direct mail campaign and yet 40% of its success is riding on using the right list, be careful. Don't rent the cheapest mailing list. Rent the best.

List Formats—Lists can be formatted in a number of ways. The most common and least expensive is 4-up Cheshire labels. Printed on computer paper with 44 to a page, these labels require a Cheshire machine to affix them to the mailing piece. Most mailings over a couple of hundred should be done with this format since your mailing house will affix them inexpensively.

Pressure-sensitive or peel-off labels that your staff can affix could be used for small-sized mailings. Pressure-sensitive labels cost slightly more than 4-up Cheshire labels, but they don't require machinery to stick them on the envelope.

Lists can also come on magnetic tape. This format is most often used for very large mailings or for computer personalization of the mailing piece. Costs are also greater than 4-up Cheshire.

List Testing—What happens if a list has 10,000 names but you know you need to do a sample test before committing to a mailing that large? Ask what their minimum test quantity is and request an "N*th* select." If the test quantity is 2,500 for a universe of 10,000, an N*th* select will print out every fourth name on the list (N*th* = universe quantity divided by test quantity). The N*th* select assures you that your sample will be representative of the entire list so you receive reliable results.

Also request that the broker keep a duplicate file of the names you ordered for the test and each subsequent mailing. Then when you request the list again, the names you're already mailed to can be removed.

Results—A year ago, a Michigan G.P. mailed 8,200 pieces promoting

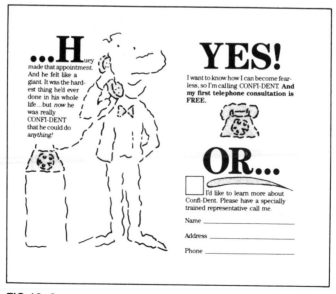

FIG 16–6.

☐ Direct Mail Tips

Here are two tips to increase the responses from direct mail authority H. Gordon Lewis:[2]

1. *Color vs. black and white*: You'd be surprised how many times using color in a direct mail piece doesn't outpull black and white enough to justify the extra cost. Or how full color doesn't output a less costly two- or three-color package.

2. *Motivators*: Different motivators work differently on different target groups. The two main motivators in this age of skepticism are guilt and greed. Sometimes a testimonial works better with status seekers. Sometimes cold, hard facts outpull everything. How do you know which pulls best? You test or rely on the expertise of someone who has.

---

his family practice. Initial mailing results: 17 responses, or 0.2%. Cost: $3,188. Net loss: $1,054. Then by using a list broker, he better targeted his prospective patients as those 25 years old and older and tested homeowners vs. renters. New results: 5,150 pieces mailed with 41 responses—a 0.7% response rate. Cost: $1,905. Net profit: $5,844. Renters responded slightly better than homeowners because of the high turnover in the area. "I used a shotgun approach in the first mailing," the physician explained. "Using a rifle not only makes a lot more sense, it makes for a much better response."

☐ LOOK TO LONGER LETTERS

In spite of what you may have heard, in direct mail a longer letter or other copy often outpulls a shorter one. Tests have shown that a two-page letter expanded to four pages will almost invariably increase response.

This is true even though many people read direct mail with one eye on the wastebasket.

Here are three major reasons why.

- Long letters can impress and convince readers. The more you say and explain, the more valuable your services are seen to be.
- You can get readers who just scan the letter to come back and read it by using graphic highlighting, sizzling subheads, and eye-catching indentations.

■ You allow for more development of your message. In a long letter, you can often do a more complete job.

So long letters create an impression of importance and authority, but only if the copy continues to interest and excite.

Tactic—One question many practitioners ask is, "Will anyone read such a long letter?" The answer is that some people will and some won't. Those who won't will probably skim the letter. So make sure you break up the copy with plenty of subhead titles.

Here are two ways to make sure your longer letter does indeed work well. First, put the emphasis on the prospective patient you're writing to and write about him or her. Use plenty of "you" copy, and let the readers know that you're interested in their needs and concerns. This makes for more interesting reading to them.

Second, stress benefits. If the service is a health checkup, stress the benefit of being free from worry. If you're promoting your background, emphasize how they'll feel confident about you.

Bottom Line—No one can give all the reasons why longer copy works. But more and more professionals are discovering that long letters get more response. That's the bottom line.

P.S.—People will read a long letter *only* if it's interesting. Length alone isn't sufficient. And don't forget the most read part of the letter—the P.S.

☐ FOUR DIRECT MAIL TECHNIQUES THAT WORK WONDERS

Recent studies of direct mail results[3] confirm what experts have been saying for years: Certain direct response techniques work wonders. The findings:

	RESPONSE RATE, %	
TECHNIQUE	WITHOUT TECHNIQUE	WITH TECHNIQUE
Teaser copy on outside of envelope or self-mailer	0.9	1.1
Including a reprint of an article	1.1	1.6
Including a letter of endorsement (check state regulations for restrictions)	0.98	1.3
Offering a premium	0.8	0.95

☐ *THE PRACTICE BUILDER'S* FIVE RULES OF DIRECT MAIL

Rule 1—To find out what combination of elements works in your direct mail, you must test them. Experiment with what's offered, benefits stressed, mailing lists, pricing if mentioned, copy on the outside of the envelope, envelopes vs. self-mailers, printed postal marks vs. stamps vs. metering.

Concentrate on the big ideas, usually the first six elements listed above. How else can you discover a bigger idea if you don't test for one against a standard?

Rule 2—After you've tested to find out what's working, continue testing. The market is forever in motion—people's buying habits change with seasons, with more competitors, with the economy, with new developments, and so on. To keep tabs on the market, keep testing.

Rule 3—Test again.

Rule 4—And then, test one more time.

Rule 5—Afterward—well, there is no afterward since you should never stop testing. No matter how limited the budget, test another variable against your standard to improve your results.

Follow-up: When you've developed at least two packages, test 1,000 or 2,000 of each, strict coding each piece to track their respective responses.

On a Roll—When the winner appears—the one with a return that's more than 10% better than the other—roll it out. But mail no more than five times as many as you sent in the first test to see if your results are replicated. Sometimes they're not because of sampling error, and an error on a full rollout of 15,000 to 25,000 pieces is more costly than you would care to dream. If the second mailing is profitable, roll out fully. You're now safe.

But remember at each step to continue testing.

REFERENCES

1. Stone B: *Successful Direct Marketing Methods*, ed 2. Chicago, Crain Books, 1984, p 28.
2. Lewis HL: *How to Make Your Advertising Twice as Effective at Half the Cost.* Chicago, Nelson Hall, Inc, 1979, p 117.
3. Huey C: Four direct mail techniques that work. *Direct Response*, February 1985, p 3 (Infomat Inc, 2550 Hawthorne Blvd, Torrance, CA, 90505).

■ CHAPTER 17
Newspaper Ads, Radio, TV, And Other Media: How To Create Tasteful And Response-Oriented Promotions

☐ WHEN TO RUN ADS IN NEWSPAPERS

Local newspapers and shoppers offer a repetitive medium that is best for generalists and for specialists who are needed infrequently or by only a small percentage of the population. Ophthalmology and psychiatry are examples of the fields that fall under this rule.

Repetition is needed because your ad must be in front of prospective patients' eyes as they enter the market. Then the use of one-time direct mail can effectively supplement and reinforce the newspaper and shopper ads.

Where Are You?—Location within the market you serve also has a bearing on the medium you choose. Big urban practices in major markets can buy regional newspaper, radio, or TV ads and make them work because, inasmuch as the practices are centrally located, they can draw from all over.

Practices in small, isolated markets can do the same at much less cost. But suburban practices in one corner of a market or small urban practices can't afford the major, high-priced media of their area. In those cases, the cost of the mass media precludes them. When those practices are ones that are needed on an ongoing basis by people or serve a large percentage of the population, they would be better advised to use direct mail. It's targetable, affordable, and can generate immediate response.

Practitioners are occasionally tempted to run in two newspapers instead of just one, as if they then might spread the risk? "Don't do it," advises ad legend David Ogilvy.[1] Concentrate what money you have in one medium, running your message sufficiently often so that the repetition makes it effective. Remember: The later repetitions bring more responses than the initial ones.

Which Newspaper?—The question then becomes which newspaper to use in markets served by more than one. What works in one newspaper may not work in another. Why? Because they're geared to different socioeconomic groups. For instance in New York, *The Daily Mirror* delivers the blue-collar trade, while *The New York Times* caters to the white-collar crowd. So you don't try to reach construction workers in *The Times*, and you don't place an elegant carriage-trade ad in *The Mirror*.

Evaluate the competing media carefully. Ask for their reader demographics—particularly income, education, male-female split, age, and zip code distribution. Then compare.

Beware: One investigation showed 10% of one newspaper's circulation was at race tracks; the newspaper was bought just for its racing sheet. That's 10% of the readership a physician might have paid to reach that would never have seen his or her ad.

☐ PAID OR FREE NEWSPAPERS?

Controversy has raged for years over whether paid subscription newspapers deliver prospects better than free newspapers. Some say paid subscriptions indicate greater interest and therefore generate greater response. But the studies are inconclusive.

However, here are three conclusions you *can* take to the bank. (1) Free newspapers delivered to the home produce far more response than those available for picking up at stores or even those stuffed in with groceries. Avoid those not home delivered. (2) Even though circulation of home-delivered free papers may be high, readership is very low. But if the circulation is high enough, a free paper may then be a good response-producing vehicle. Only testing can tell. (3) Circulation figures of free newspapers are unaudited, unlike that of most of the paid newspapers. Therefore, don't expect the publisher's figures to be accurate. Assume that they're greatly inflated.

☐ AD ANALYSIS: REACHING MOM

The ad shown in Figure 17–1 will catch the eye of any mother who has a child who suffers from asthma. The photograph of the youngster coupled with the headline tell the whole story. But even those who just glance at the ad may pick up the more subtle message

☐ Is Color In Ads Worth It?

In newspaper advertising for professional services, the color black alone is almost always sufficient. Only in those unusual cases when colorful products are shown is the extra cost of additional color justified. Remember: Black is the strongest color.

---

conveyed by the bolder portion of the headline: "Asthma Relieved."

Put this ad in the life-style section or TV section of the newspaper, and the response will leave this practice trying to catch its breath.

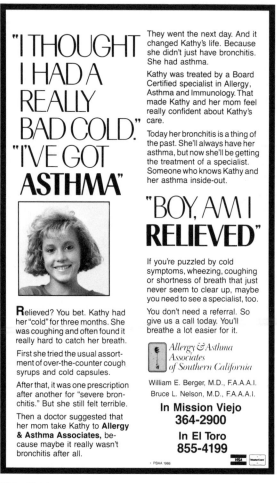

FIG 17–1.

☐ LOCATION DETERMINES AD SUCCESS

In newspaper advertising, effectiveness depends on where your ad is located in the paper. The best tactic is to locate it next to related editorial material and in the section that the audience you wish to reach looks. Different sections have distinctly different readerships. Sports reach a 90% male audience. Editorials reach the few civic-minded readers. The general news readership is 60% to 70% male. Wednesday's or Thursday's food section and the life-styles section are read by women.

Overall, newspapers are poor choices for reaching younger people. Today newspaper readership is older—40+ because those 18 to 34 years old use other media, particularly television, much more than the local paper. If you're still sold on newspapers and want to reach younger readers, test your ad in one section most read by younger people—the comic page. In fact, it's the most read section of the paper and is seen by both kids and adults.

Another Choice—Another wise location to reach a complete cross section of ages and one with high readership is to have your ad appear in the separate weekly TV listings. Included with the weekend paper, it stays around the house all week long. Good position: Front inside cover, back cover, and within the Sunday night listings. Sunday draws the largest television audiences.

Within the regular news sections, the position on the page and within the section also affects the ad's success. "All newspaper ads should be placed on the top half of the page," advises Dr. Peter Fernandez, president of Practice Motivation International.[2] Work for increased noticeability by requiring that the newspaper run your ad on the upper half of the page that readers scan first.

Fernandez suggests that in general "the ad should be placed on page two or three of the first section of the newspaper if possible." Sometimes these ad positions carry a premium rate. If the ad is good, it's almost always worth it, since prospective patients can't respond if they don't see your ad.

☐ HOW BIG SHOULD A NEWSPAPER AD BE?

Answer 1—Big enough to communicate your message. If the concept is familiar, less space is needed. But if the subject matter is complex

☐ Best Newspaper Sections

When you run a newspaper ad, the question is always in which section should it appear. Why? Because placement can affect your results by up to 1,000%. Here's where 212 high-volume newspaper advertisers place their ads for the big payback:

TARGET MARKET	SUNDAY LOCATION	DAILY LOCATION
Affluent males	Business	Business
Middle-income males	Sports	Sports
Affluent females	Business	Women's
Middle-income females	Main news	Women's
Affluent males and females	Business	Main news
Middle-income males and females	Main news or TV Section	Main news or TV section

Also request a righthand page, upper-righthand placement as far forward in the section as possible. But in the TV section, request placement among the Sunday listings because that's the day of the most television viewing. Requests aren't always honored unless you pay a premium for a preferred section. But always request.

---

or unfamiliar (radial keratotomy), or if it's one in which fears have to be allayed (cosmetic surgery), a bigger ad should be bought.

Answer 2—Big enough to be noticed. Many practitioners buy as small a space as they can and then cram it full to get their money's worth. As a consequence, the ad gets buried beneath an avalanche of similar-sized advertisements and goes unnoticed. Also, because of the crowded, cluttered appearance, the ad looks thoroughly unprofessional and communicates that image about the practitioner.

Solution—Buy enough space to communicate, enough space to set yourself apart from the pile of other ads, and enough space to convey a good professional image.

☐ DON'T USE YOUR *YELLOW PAGES* AD IN THE NEWSPAPER

Yellow Pages and newspaper ads reach different audiences and consequently can't be interchanged freely. In the *Yellow Pages* your readers have already decided they need the services of someone in your profession. Their big question: Why you? The headline, copy, and graphics should all be geared to answer that question head-on.

Different Readership—In newspapers, readers haven't qualified their interest as they have in the *Yellow Pages*. So the first job for your ad to do is to tell them what you do; then why they should choose you. Both can be accomplished in the ad, but usually with a different headline, body copy, and graphics than those that appear in your *Yellow Pages* ad.

Also in newspapers, ads tend to be a bit "noisier" to overcome the intense commercial clutter there. This affects the ad's size, style, and flavor.

So for best results, use different ads to address these two different purposes.

☐ AD ANALYSIS: THE BEST IN SIGHT

If newspaper ads in general are a bit noisier, then an effective ad needs to speak up—not scream, not shout, just speak loudly enough to get attention. As seen in Figure 17–2, the short, attention-grabbing question, "Fading Vision?" reinforced by a very effective series of fading photographs leaves no question about the problem and the benefit the ad promises.

Although the headline is large enough to demand attention, even on a crowded newspaper page, notice that this ad isn't cluttered or crowded. That gives it a professional look that will set it apart from the other competing ads that surround it.

This ad will also work beautifully and is so appropriate for newspapers because of that medium's aging readers. The ad doesn't make outlandish claims ("You'll find specialists who *may* be able to restore your sight . . . ."), but it does promote the practice's high technology.

The benefit of no hospitalization and free screening will also appeal to the target market.

All in all, this is an ad with vision.

☐ RADIO—THE WINNING WAY

Radio advertising can be a good vehicle. Mainly because it's an *intrusive* medium. That means the audience doesn't need to decide whether to read your ad as they do with newspapers, shoppers, or direct mail. Instead, you reach those who are listening to a station, and they hear the message without any decision or action on their part. This intrusiveness generates a higher awareness than media where a choice is involved.

But it is very possible for the inexperienced advertiser to buy the wrong amounts of time aired at the wrong times and on the wrong station.

The Right Station—Different stations, of course, have different listenerships. In fact, many have different audiences at different times of the day. The right station with the right stuff is determined by the

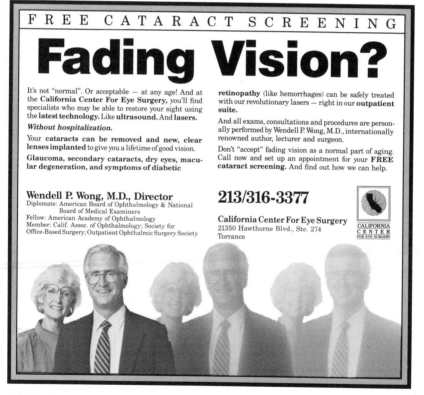

FIG 17–2.

definition of your target market, whether that station reaches that market, and then whether the station delivers to your target economically—without the waste of reaching large numbers of people who have no interest in your services.

Choosing the right station needn't be complex. First, define your target. For example, assume you want to reach females aged 25 to 49 years old. You would ask each likely station in your area for their *latest* Arbitron rating sheet, which gives their overall ratings as well as the specific ratings for your target market.

Trustworthy Numbers—Arbitron is to radio what Neilsen is to television: the independent auditor of radio station audiences. Theirs are the only figures you can trust. Arbitron is a subscription service, so you need to get the ratings free from the stations you're considering. They should be happy to give them out—unless they're too embarrassed.

Then get the station's advertising rate card. Take their cost per 60-second spot and divide it by the average number of thousand of listeners *in your target group*. Ignore the rest of the audience. What this computation gives you is the average cost of delivering your message to 1,000 of your prime prospective patients.

With this efficiency measure you can now rank stations and find out which ones are the best buys—the ones with the lowest cost per thousand (CPM) for your targets. Cost per thousand is the only meaningful statistic in determining how to buy radio—*not* the actual cost per spot.

The Responsive Station—Even though two stations may deliver the same target at the same CPM efficiency, they may still have different response rates. Why? Because the two groups of listeners can differ psychographically, i.e., by life-style, tastes, interests, and the like.

By and large, the more interactive the station format, the better the response rate. News or talk stations do very well. Background music stations don't. People only listen to such elevator music with a quarter of their attention. Country delivers a less responsive audience than does a mellow rock station with the same demographics. Tactic: After the quantitative analysis, further rank stations qualitatively.

The Right Amount—One station is rarely enough to buy. With so many stations in every market, most stations can claim only a small percentage of your target market. Hence you need to buy time on more than one station. Determine how many stations not only by your budget, but also by the goal of your effort. The bigger the goal, the larger the number of listeners you need.

But if you have a limited budget for airwaves promotion, it's better to concentrate on one station—preferably a large, network station—than buying less repetition on two or more smaller stations.

The Right Time—Especially important is the number of spots and their times of airing. Morning drive time is not only the most expensive but also the most responsive. People seem willing to take care of life's needs when they're fresh and have energy—not at the end of the day. Weekend spots perform poorly. Everyone's too busy relaxing.

A study has also shown that responses increase dramatically if the spots are aired when the office is open and therefore listeners can call immediately to book an appointment—before they forget the name, the number, or your convincing reasons for seeing you. Also, if you're promoting extended hours, advertise them at times just prior and during those hours. Response jumps dramatically.

Therefore, most practices do well when they run a minimum of two morning drive spots Monday through Friday, requesting that the station air them between 7 A.M. and 9 A.M. Other times of the day are less responsive, but they help boost response of the morning spots. If the budget permits, buy another one or two midday spots (10 A.M. to 3 P.M.) and even one or two evening drive spots (3 P.M. to 7 P.M.). Forget 7 P.M. to 6 A.M.

Schedule 9 out of the next 12 weeks with the ads not aired every fourth week. This schedule buys you about the same payback as a continuous run. Unless you commit to that amount of repetition and that weight of media, the results are doomed.

Unfortunately, that's the sorry lesson learned by some professionals who run 60-second "here-and-gone" spots. But the average listener needs to hear a message between *five and seven* times before reacting. So when you play the radio game, buy repetition, and buy enough listeners—or don't play the game at all.

Three Other Radio Tips—When you've decided on the stations, ignore the rate card. It's only there to convince the naive to pay a higher rate. Negotiate hard to reduce costs 15% to 50%. Remember: This is a very quantity-sensitive buy.

Second, the most expensive times of year are the times of greatest demand: Christmas, summer, and during important elections. Softest rate times: January through March.

Third, forget 30-second spots. You need enough time to catch the listeners' attention, develop a message, and convince prospective patients to call. You must repeat your phone number two or three times as well. Thirty-second spots don't allow enough time to explain and

☐ Demand A 'Make Good'

Because radio and television transmissions are highly technical, at times your spot may not air properly. Part or all of it may not run, or it may run inappropriately. If this happens, you're entitled to a repeat of the spot that's run correctly, and at a time that gives you the same exposure or ratings as the original would have had. Insist on it because you won't get it otherwise.

convince. They were created so that television advertisers could use the soundtrack from their 30-second TV commercials and not have the additional production costs of creating radio spots twice as long as their TV messages. So stick with 60-second messages that only cost 117% of 30-second ones.

If you have a *large budget* but don't want to get involved in negotiating for the broadcast time, try a media buying service. These groups buy in bulk and buy with wisdom. And the media pays their commission so there's no extra cost to you.

Results—Physician M.P. targeted 25- to 49-year-old females in blue-collar or clerical positions. He had two 60-second spots created by a specialty ad agency and bought two mellow rock/middle-of-the-road stations reaching 38% of his target market. On each station he bought two morning drive, one midday, and one evening drive spots Monday to Thursday. Monthly cost: $1,800. Cost of running 9 weeks out of 12: $5,400. Results: 92 calls, 56 additional patients averaging $785 each. Total income: $43,960. Return on investment in 180 days: 814%.

"I'd been on radio before, but it wasn't as productive. I think the difference this time is the spots are more convincing and also the number of spots I bought. My first time on radio I didn't buy enough because I was trying to conserve money. But obviously that wasn't the right way."

☐ TV IS PRIME FOR ONLY A FEW PRACTITIONERS

Everyone talks about the power of TV. Your response is greatest—but so are your costs. In all except the smallest markets, practitioners can only afford to buy time during the daytime when prices are cheaper. With prime time (8 to 11 P.M.), early fringe (5 to 8 P.M.) and late fringe (11 P.M. to 1 A.M.), you can reach working people, but the costs are universally prohibitive, particularly in large markets.

So that leaves daytime for the average practitioner. And who watches then? Senior citizens, the unemployed, the few housewives left, the ill and the injured. All except the unemployed are good prospects for some kind of medical practice. Still production costs tend to keep most docs on the sidelines in this game.

Special Circumstances—Television can make sense in very small broadcast markets or for very large practices or, as discussed in Chapter 10, for a group of physicians in a cooperative venture who pool their resources to advertise in expensive mass media. Even large practices or cooperative ventures should be in a medical field with broad applications so that the use of television is justified by the large numbers of prospective patients reached.

For appropriate groups of physicians able to afford it, dollars spent on great television advertising buy more prospects than the same money would buy in direct mail or newspapers. And TV works faster because it has a unique immediacy and excitement that produces results in greater numbers than any other medium.

But remember, the start-up costs are high. And the quality of respondents is usually inferior to those generated by mail or print media. This, however, can be adjusted by fine-tuning the TV spot to appeal to just the right prospective patient.

Immediate Responses—In TV, use a minimum of a 30-second spot. When you run it, you'll immediately get responses, so be ready with a number of phone lines. Busy signals cause a significant loss of business.

When a prospective patient calls, not only book the appointment, but take their address and phone number, and mail them a brochure right away. This reduces no-shows by reinforcing the points made in the commercial. Make sure the brochure strongly reiterates those one or two points made in the spot. Also, if they don't show, call within 15 minutes to reiterate the benefits, and reschedule the appointments.

Test your commercial at different times of the day on different stations until you find your best returns. Most of the time, this means avoiding cable television because of its low number of viewers in general and much lower number of qualified prospects than in the market in particular.

The Spot's Structure—In your commercial, follow this outline:

1. Statement of benefits or a problem (5 to 10 seconds)
2. Dramatization (10 to 20 seconds)
3. Telephone number and/or address (5 to 10 seconds)

It's an expensive game, but a profitable one. And it's not for the weakhearted, so consider doing it in a group. In any case, when advertising on television, always use professional help. It's too risky for the novice alone.

☐ BEWARE OF CITY MAGAZINES

Those slick, often chic, city magazines like *New York* and *Los Angeles Magazine* are popping up in every area with middle-income to affluent market segments. But are they a prime medium for physicians looking for upscale patients? Not if you expect immediate response. They're fine for long-term, image-building campaigns. It is best to use them in combination with a strong *Yellow Pages* display ad for optimal results.

☐ BUYING MAGAZINE SPACE

If the costs weren't so high, the *regional* issues of well-respected magazines—*Time, Newsweek, Family Circle, Sports Illustrated, Reader's Digest, Ladies Home Journal*—would be an ideal media for many professionals.

At times, there is space available at deep discounts. These 11th hour availabilities, called "remnant buys," arise when someone cancels an ad or the space just isn't selling as usual. Price is very negotiable, but you must have an ad already prepared, ready to be rushed into the gap.

Get in touch with the magazines' reps in your area to let them know of your interest in those remnant buys.

☐ MULTIPLE SHOPPER ADS

If you're running ads in local shoppers or any print medium, every time the ad is given poor placement—toward the back or on a lefthand page in the gutter (next to the inside fold)—you can expect responses to fall. It's simply because fewer people will see your ad when it is given those placements. But unfortunately, you can't ensure a better position unless you buy the front or back covers.

Instead, consider running multiple ads in the same issue. Dispersed properly, three ads seem to work optimally. These almost guarantee that at least one of them will be read. And chances are more than one will be read. So repetition will work in your favor.

If one insertion per week is already working, test three.

☐ OTHER MEDIA: NEW AFFORDABLE MEDIUM NOW AVAILABLE

The third largest movie-house chain in the country, American Multi Cinema (AMC), recently formed a new subsidiary, National Cinema Network (NCN), to put local advertisers on at the nearest of their 1,100 movie screens across the country. That means that sole practitioners can now promote to a captive audience in a very localized area—and do it affordably. Here's how it works.

You contact the local NCN rep, AMC theater, or call 1–800–558–1539. Reps are presently based in Florida, Washington, D.C., Detroit, Kansas City/St. Louis, Denver, Houston, Dallas, Phoenix, Los Angeles, and San Jose/San Francisco, but each covers a large area. And more are on the way.

You contract to have them make a slide of your promotion that is flashed at the local theater for 10 seconds prior to the start of the film. Music provided by the theater accompanies the slides.

During the typical 13-week run, your slide will be exposed 250 to 500 times depending on the number of screens in the theater. That's a lot of repetition to an audience attentively waiting for the film to start.

Benefits—This medium works best in the following manner. When you primarily target lower-middle to middle income 18- to 34-year-olds, these spots give you good coverage. Also, since 60% of the patrons come from within 5 to 7 miles away, you can target geographically.

Use your slide best to increase response to your other promotions such as your *Yellow Pages* and other ads. When they've seen your ad projected on screen, they'll recognize it in the *Yellow Pages* or other media, which is why you should use similar copy and graphics in all the ads.

The program cost depends on the average attendance by the theater. Typically, this will run between $12 to $25 per week per screen. A 13-week run is the recommended minimum. Figure on another $125 or so for production of the slide by NCN's local production house.

Weaknesses—The NCN rep or the local production house will recommend a marketing strategy for the slide if you don't have one. Our recommendation: Have one ready. Don't trust their strategies, just their ability to produce a slide based upon your strategy.

REFERENCES

1. Ogilvy D: *Confessions of An Advertising Man.* New York, Atheneum Publishers, 1963, p 102.
2. Fernandez P: *Secrets of a Practice Consultant: One Thousand and One Ways to Attract New Patients.* St Petersburg, Fla, Valkyrie Publishing House, 1981, p 45.

■ CHAPTER 18
Figuring Out When You Need Professional Help And How To Find Competence

☐ UNDERSTANDING THE LIMITATIONS OF EXPERTS

All of us have limitations. The trick for the successful professional is to understand the limitations of the various experts you turn to when creating promotions. Here's a list of what *not* to expect from certain suppliers and where you'll need to supply missing information, ideas, strategies, and abilities.

- *Graphic artists*: They're not marketing people. Expect to supply the marketing strategies. Look to them only for good artistic execution of the strategy.
- *Sign companies*: Sign companies believe you should put your name and perhaps your logo on your sign. That's it. They're so design-oriented that they can't evaluate whether these elements differentiate you from competitors and motivate prospective patients to respond. Count on them to help with the size, placement, construction, perhaps the art on the sign. Don't expect effective copy or marketing concepts.
- *Printers*: Printers know printing. Not art. Not advertising. Not direct mail. Not even *good* typesetting. Certainly not marketing strategies. Expect them only to print the camera-ready materials you provide—on time and affordably.
- *Typesetters*: Typesetters have some of the same limitations— no marketing abilities. But do look for well-chosen typefaces, if you tell them the image you're trying to project, and a clean, professional layout. Remember: For results of practically any kind, you or someone else must write the copy based on sound marketing principles.

- *Yellow Pages*: You would think that of all the media, the *Yellow Pages* ad department would be able to produce outstanding—even gangbuster—*Yellow Pages* ads. Wrong, tenderfoot. Expect them only to place and print the camera-ready ad you give them. And even for that, keep your fingers crossed.
- *Newspapers, radio, television*: With these, too, there's a limitation on marketing knowledge. But they tend to be a bit more sophisticated about advertising than the *Yellow Pages*. Again, *you* must specify the marketing strategy. Expect them to know how to translate your strategy into their medium and to take particular advantage of its strengths.
- *Ad agencies*: Now we're getting even slicker. General ad agencies know how to gain attention, create a feeling, select media—but they probably don't know your profession. Again count on telling them the most effective marketing strategy and just use their fine execution. But if you want the whole kit and kaboodle taken off your hands, marketing and all, use an ad agency that has handled similar accounts. Beware: A surgeon is not the same as an ophthalmologist. A hospital is not the same as a general practitioner. Sames means same. Otherwise, you'll end up paying for their learning curve and have diminished results.

The Message—Knowing the limitations of various promotional professionals saves you lots of money and makes you lots of money. And it allows you to go to different specialists for their specialty while anticipating their inabilities.

☐ DO YOU NEED AN AD AGENCY?

Two physicians were going into private practice together. Expenses for the new office were, of course, high. So was the competition.

Partner A said, "If we're going to spend all this money launching the practice, let's make sure our promotion really pays—let's hire a good agency." Partner B disagreed, "I think I can make up all the ads. I'm pretty creative and good with words. Besides, look at all the money we'll save."

Feeling a surge of anger, the first partner raised his voice. "We're going to have to spend $8,000 in the *Yellow Pages* alone, and you want to save a few bucks by doing the ad yourself, or having those $3.35-an-hour *Yellow Pages* cartoonists do it. What do you know about advertising? You've never done an ad before. And now you want me to gamble my money on your advertising ability?"

With hackles raised, the second partner answered, "Look, we don't have that much money to afford a fancy ad agency. Besides, the people at the *Yellow Pages* do these ads all the time."

The argument continued along those same lines. Then the conversation ended and so did the partnership. It reverted to a facility-sharing arrangement with both practitioners promoting on their own and therefore competing against each other.

Garbage In . . .—The computer adage also applies to advertising. If you put garbage in the media, you invariably get garbage out. Unfortunately, much homemade advertising is just that. For example, look through your local *Yellow Pages*. How many practitioners have used their names as the headline as if that will bring anyone in the office. It's worthless. In a word—garbage.

But if you turn to a specialist, make sure he or she is really a specialist. An ad agency must specialize in professional services in general. They need to show you they're fully familiar with your field and have produced successfully ads for someone very much like you. They should also utilize proper testing methods—like A/B splits that'll tell them which of two strategies works best.

In newspapers, an A/B split means that two different ads with different phone numbers or extensions for tracking are run in the same edition, with each ad appearing in half the papers. In direct mail, it means two different packages are sent; half the households receive one, and half receive the other. A/B split testing means you needn't guess which strategy works best with a given market. You know.

The Difference—Using techniques such as A/B splits, a specialty agency can create an ad that outpulls one produced by an amateur. It will also outperform an ad created by those who don't specialize and don't test. That includes the *Yellow Pages* art department, the newspaper, radio and TV stations, and even general ad agencies.

And the real difference? Not an ad that's just twice as effective. Or three or four times. But one that achieves up to 10 or even 20 times the response rate. In the partnership mentioned earlier, that could have meant a difference of the *Yellow Pages* producing $4,000, or producing $90,000.

☐ HIRING A MARKETING FIRM

Family practitioner C.C. walked into a Massachusetts public relations firm to see if they could help him generate new patients. Their answer: "Of course." The program: Arranging two talk shows and two articles in the local weekly newspaper. His cost: $3,000. His loss: $3,000. His problem: Not understanding that public relations like this must be long range if it's to bring in the patients he wants.

Another New Englander, obstetrician/gynecologist L.D., called a local ad agency with the same request. Their answer: "Of course." Their program: Local name recognition advertising on two small radio stations. His cost: $4,350. His loss: $2,170. His problem: Not understanding that the budget was too small to meet the goal and that the agency knew it, but took his money anyway.

When the Solution Is the Problem—Doctors approach marketing firms in good faith—and perhaps with some naïveté—with cries for help and money to spend. But here's what goes wrong.

First, if you go only to a public relations firm, then the answer to any marketing question automatically is public relations, even though there may be 15 better avenues.

Second, the problem is often not giving the firm enough resources to work with. Except for certain direct mailings, any promotion requires repetition as has been said repeatedly in this book. There's a minimum expenditure necessary to make a go of the promotion. If you can't or won't spend it, then you're better off not playing the game at all. Because the agency will take your money even if the meager amount you're willing to spend automatically dooms the effort.

Third, the firm may not know what they're doing. And since the average practitioner may know even less, they become easy prey. And practice management firms are often guilty of giving marketing advice without any formal education or experience in marketing. They may know lots about personnel, finance, time management, office layouts, and such, but if you ask them for their marketing credentials, all you'll get is foot shuffling.

How To Choose The Right Firm—It's obvious from C.C.'s experience that there's a danger in going to a firm that specializes in only one kind of promotion. First, make sure it's the answer you want. A better strategy: Go to a firm that provides an array of marketing services.

Then thoroughly check the marketing credentials of your candidates. Be merciless. Do they have M.B.A.s in marketing? *Any* degrees in marketing? Have they dealt with practices similar to yours? In similar target markets? What works with one type of prospective patient only sometimes works with others.

Can they give you hard numbers to not only show the number of new patients generated, but also how much each patient spent on the average with the practitioner? Can they give you the return on investment that each of their different types of promotion has historically generated? Can they give you at least five "I swear by this firm" referrals?

And what's the first thing they'll do? If it's not analyzing the market, they don't know marketing. Even if you're inexperienced in marketing, you can still tell the soft shuffles from the firm, confident marches. Avoid those that lack hard numbers. And you'll avoid those that will practice with your money. Only a firm that stands up to this kind of scrutiny is worth your consideration.

☐ AD AGENCY FEE SURVEY

What do ad agencies charge? Many professionals would answer, "A lot." Others would say, "It doesn't matter as long as they make money for the practice." These remarks point out that that the fee charged is only one element in choosing an agency. The most important factor is their track record with similar accounts.

Still, it's helpful to know how much agencies charge in general. So *The Practice Builder* conducted a price survey of 23 agencies that had produced ads or other materials for at least one practitioner. They ranged from a one-person shop to a medium-sized agency with over 20 employees. Only those agencies that had a full range of professional capabilities were included—those with writing, art, marketing, and media in-house. They also had to be in business at least 3 years. No freelancers were surveyed. Just full-service agencies staffed by professionals.

Within this group, fees didn't vary according to the size of the agency. But when *The Practice Builder* checked with agencies of more than 25 employees or $10 million in billings, prices jumped significantly. This is not the kind of firm professionals often turn to for help since they often end up as the little fish in a big pond with the copywriter-in-training assigned to their account. For that reason, large firms were not included in the survey.

Neither were "canned" ad programs where the ads created only promote the profession, and the company slaps the doctor's name at the bottom almost as an afterthought. Only those agencies producing individualized campaigns were investigated. All prices include "camera-ready" artwork—meaning the materials are ready to send to the printer or the *Yellow Pages* directory. Printing is not included in the prices shown.

Use this data to make sure you're not being overcharged. Here's what *The Practice Builder* discovered:

PROJECT	RANGE, $	MEAN, $
Marketing-based logo, letterhead envelope, and business card	750–4,250	1,625
Practice brochure/direct mailer 8 1/2 × 15 in., 3-fold, 8 panels, 2 sides	1,900–5,400	2,875
Yellow Pages ad: 2 columns × 1/2-page high	500–3,000	1,000
Yellow Pages ad: 1/2-page horizontal	750–4,000	1,450
Three newspaper ads: 3 columns × 6 in.	1,350–5,000	1,900
Two 60-second radio spots including minimal production	2,000–5,000	2,675
One 30-second TV spot including storyboard and production on videotape	6,800–14,500	9,300
Advertising action plan: complete analysis and planning document for budgets over $35,000	750–5,000	2,600

■ GLOSSARY

A/B split testing. See "split run."

Advertising. A nonpersonal presentation usually directed to a large number of people intended to interest them in the sponsor's product or services.

Agate line. A unit of measurement in classified advertising equal to the column width by 1/14 in. deep.

Airbrushing. A technique using a small gun that sprays paint or pigment that is used to create illustrations or to retouch photographs, for example, to remove a facial blemish.

Arbitron. The independent auditor of radio station audiences.

Art (also artwork). Illustrative material including both drawings and photographs used in promotional materials and other printed matter.

Audit Bureau of Circulations (ABC). The organization sponsored by magazine publishers, agencies, and advertisers to obtain accurate circulation figures.

Author's corrections/alterations. Changes made to the proofs of typeset material that are not printer's typographical errors. Such AAs are an unnecessary expense that can be avoided by careful editing in the initial stages.

Bait and switch. An unethical, illegal tactic in which one attractive product or service is advertised although the advertiser has no intention of selling it or has it in such short supply that the effect is the same. Instead, the intention is to convince a prospect to switch to and buy a costlier product or service.

Black and white. Printing done in one color usually with black ink on white paper. To be differentiated from two-, three-, four-color printing.

Bleed. An illustration or photograph that is printed so that part of it continues off the page, leaving no margin.

Body copy. The main text in a printed piece as opposed to headlines and other display matter.

Body type. The lighter, smaller typeface in which text is typically set compared with display faces. Usually type that is 14 points in size or smaller.

Boldface. Type that is heavier and thicker than text type (such as the entries in this glossary).

Bullet. A small solid circle used as a graphic device to set off paragraphs or placed before items in a list to attract attention.

Buying space. Buying the right to insert an advertisement in a given medium such as a magazine or newspaper. With electronic media, the comparable term is "buying time."

Camera-ready. An ad, brochure, or other material that has been typeset and laid out and its artwork has been finished so the printer can reproduce it without any further alteration.

Circulation. The number of people that a publication or medium reaches.

Closing. The final step in a presentation in which the prospect is asked for a decision.

Closing date. The publication deadline for submitting material for a particular issue.

Coated paper. Paper having a surface coating that produces a smooth finish.

Color separation. The process of separating a full-color photograph or illustration into the primary colors, which will permit it to be printed in color rather than black and white.

Column inch. A unit of measure that is one column wide and 1 in. deep and primarily used in buying advertising space in newspapers and magazines.

Composite print. A print of a television commercial complete with audio and visual.

Composition. Typesetting.

Comprehensive. A layout created to show the actual size, colors, and other specifics to demonstrate how the ad will appear.

Controlled circulation. Publications with circulations that are limited by the publisher to a particular readership.

Cooperative advertising. A program in which advertising costs are shared between a group of advertisers who benefit from the advertisement.

Copy. (1) The text of an advertisement. (2) Any material to be used in the production of a periodical.

Copywriter. A person who creates advertisements and writes the text for them.

Copywriting. The creation of an ad and particularly the full text of what it is to say.

Cost per thousand. Used to compare media costs, it is a computation of the cost to reach a thousand viewers, readers, or prospects. Usually denoted as CPM.

Coupon. A sales promotion technique that offers a discount from the regular price or fee.

CPM. See cost per thousand.

Crop. To trim portions of an illustration or photograph to make it a desired size or to remove unessential parts of it.

Demographics. The various characteristics, such as age, income, and social class, that distinguish a particular group. Also refers to the type of audience a publication or program reaches.

Direct mail advertising. A type of direct response advertising in which promotional materials are mailed to prospects.

Direct response advertising (also direct marketing). Advertising that includes an offer to which members of the audience can respond by calling, mailing, or otherwise contacting an office directly.

Display advertising. In newspapers, ads other than those in the classified section. In the *Yellow Pages*, ads other than the in-column listings.

Display type. Type that is typically larger than 18 points and in a distinctive boldface that is used in headlines and other placements to gain attention.

Double spread. Two facing pages used as a single unbroken advertisement.

Dummy. A sketched or mocked up sample of a pamphlet, direct mailer, book, or other material to indicate its final appearance and size.

Font. A complete assortment of type of one size and face, including caps, lowercase, numerals, and punctuation marks.

Format. The size, shape, style, and appearance of an ad, brochure, newsletter, or other publication.

Four-color.   A process using a press with plates that print the black and three primary colors to reproduce the full range of intermediate and other colors.

Frequency rates.   Advertising rates determined by the number of insertions contracted within a period of time. Such rates typically include a frequency discount.

Galley proofs.   Sheets of typeset copy prepared for proofreading.

Gutter.   The inner margin of facing pages in a publication.

Hairlines.   Extremely thin rules—lines—used to box copy or for other graphic uses.

Halftone.   A photoengraving process that reduces a photograph (or other continuous tone image) to a series of minute dots that may then be printed.

Head.   A display-size caption or statement intended to gain the reader's attention and summarize an ad's contents.

Initial drop.   An oversized first letter used at the start of a paragraph to attract the reader's attention.

Insert (freestanding).   A self-contained printed advertisement of one or more pages that is inserted between the pages or sections of a newspaper or magazine.

Insertion order.   Instructions from an advertiser authorizing a publisher to print an advertisement of specified size on a given date at an agreed rate. The order is accompanied or followed by the camera-ready copy for the advertisement.

Justified type.   Setting type so that each line is exactly the same length so that the column has straight margins on both the left and right side. Compare ragged right margins.

Layout.   The total design of an advertisement or other printed matter indicating its configuration, spaces, and type specifications.

Letter shop.   A firm that not only addresses the mailing envelope but is also mechanically equipped to insert material, seal and stamp envelopes, and deliver them to the post office conforming to mailing regulations.

Linage.   The total number of lines of space occupied by one advertisement or a series of ads by an advertiser.

List broker.   In direct mail advertising, an agent who rents one-time use of a mailing list of names and addresses. The broker receives a commission from the seller for this service.

Local rates.   An advertising rate, usually lower than that for national advertisers, offered by newspapers and other media to local advertisers.

Logo or logotype.   A trademark or trade name embodied in the form of a distinctive lettering or design.

Mail order advertising.   See direct mail advertising.

Makegood.—The running of an advertisement without charge to replace a previous ad that the publisher or broadcaster agrees was poorly run or did not appear at all.

Market.   A group of people who can be identified by a common identity, interest, or problem and who have purchasing power and can be reached through some medium.

Market profile. A demographic or psychographic description of the people or households in a market.

Market research. Gathering facts needed to make marketing decisions.

Marketing. The development and efficient distribution of goods and services for chosen market segments.

Mechanical. A form of layout that shows an exact black-and-white copy of the advertisement as it will appear in print in precise position ready for the camera.

Name recognition advertising. Advertising that promotes the advantages of an advertiser and recognition of the advertiser's name. Does not include a direct response offer.

One-time rate. The classified advertising rate for a single insertion.

Open rate. See one-time rate.

Page makeup. The general appearance of a page; the arrangement of the editorial copy and advertisements.

Pica. The unit for measuring width in printing. There are 6 picas to an inch.

Position. Where your ad appears in a newspaper or magazine, or when your spot is broadcast during a radio or television program.

Preferred position. A desirable position in a publication for which the advertiser must pay a premium rate.

Prehead. A headline set in small type and placed above an ad's main headline.

Premium. A bonus item given free with the purchase of another item or service.

Press release. A news or feature story prepared by a public relations or advertising agency or other promoter for circulation by the media.

Promotion. The function of informing, persuading, and influencing the prospect's purchase decision.

Psychographics. A description of the market based on factors such as attitudes, opinions, interests, perceptions, and life-styles of the prospects who make up that market.

Publicity. The segment of public relations related to promoting a company's products or services.

Ragged right. Setting type so that the right margin is unjustified.

Rate card. A card that lists the advertising space rates of a publication based on placement, frequency, and other factors. The card also indicates circulation data and the closing dates for advertisements.

Rate protection. The length of time an advertiser is guaranteed a specific rate by a publication or station.

Release. See press release.

Retouching. The process of correcting or improving art work, especially photographs.

ROI (return on investment). In marketing, the performance ratio that determines how well a promotion has done. It is found by dividing the total income from a specific promotion by the cost of that promotion.

ROP (run of the paper). Advertising placed anywhere in a publication at the editor's option. Compare preferred position.

ROS (run of schedule). Commercials that can be scheduled at the station's discretion within a specified time period.

Rough.   A preliminary sketch of a layout showing the basic ideas and placement.

Rules.   Straight lines used to separate or box copy.

Rushes.   The first, uncorrected prints of a commercial.

Sans serif.   Typefaces that lack the short, light line projections from the top or bottom of the main stroke of a letter. Also called block lettering.

Serif.   The short, light line projecting from the top or bottom of the main stroke of a letter.

Shopper.   A weekly or less frequent publication with a newspaper format with primarily advertisements for content and delivered without charge to readers.

Short rate.   The extra rate charged to an advertiser who has not earned a previously anticipated discount given for running a specified volume of advertising.

Split run.   A facility available in some newspapers and magazines in which the advertiser can run different advertisements in alternate copies of the same issue at the same time. It is used as a pretesting method to compare the response to the two different ads published under identical conditions. Also called A/B split testing.

Spread.   (1) Two facing pages of a publication. (2) An advertisement that occupies two facing pages.

Storyboard.   The panel or series of panels with mounted rough drawings that show the action and theme of a television commercial or program.

Subhead.   A subordinate headline that is smaller than the main head but larger than the copy.

Tear sheets.   Copies of advertisements from newspapers sent to the advertiser as proof of publication.

Typeface.   The design and style of a type letter.

Type family.   A group of type designs that are variations of one basic typeface and include, for example, the italic, Roman (type that is not italic) and boldface.

■ INDEX

Stop Being The Best Kept Secret In Town!

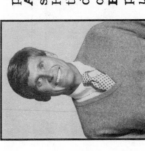

Have your promotion produced by **The Practice Builder Agency**, the most experienced specialists in the business. Having served more practitioners than anyone else -- over 1,000 doctors in all 50 states, in all types of communities -- **The Practice Builder Agency** knows your practice and your market *before you call.*

Just check the appropriate boxes on the other side and a senior specialist in your type of practice will call you to explore your needs. Then he'll explain how **The Practice Builder Agency** can fulfill your needs within a prudent budget. Of course, there's no obligation to inquire.

Simply complete the other side of this form and mail or call today!

Now More Patient Boosting Strategies...And Your Own Personal Marketing Advisor

Would you like all the newest patient-generating ideas, created by the only Marketing Think-Tank for Physicians in the nation? Plus, your own personal marketing advisor to help you implement the perfect marketing strategies just for your practice?

Now you can...because they're available from **THE PRACTICE BUILDER**, the award-winning marketing pros who created all the strategies and tactics in this book. And now you can receive their newest strategies *before* they come out years later in book form...and well before your colleagues can use them.

Plus, get your own personal advisor with an M.B.A. in Marketing to show you how to custom-fit these strategies to *your* practice. To *your* community. With eight, intensive 15-minute consultations each year...up to two full hours (a $300 value!)

SPECIAL SAVINGS FOR PURCHASERS OF THIS BOOK: *Save Half-Off the regular membership price.* ☞